Pickard's Manual of Operative Dentistry

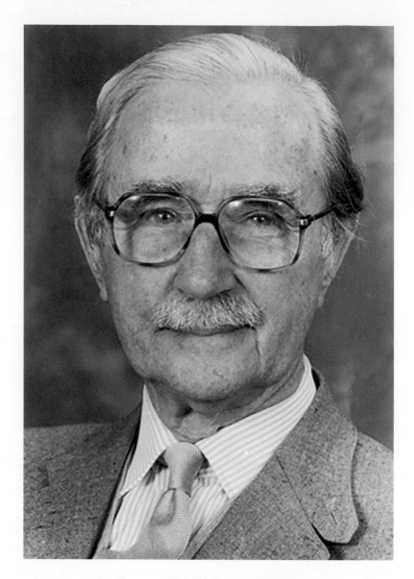

Professor HM Pickard 1909–2002

Pickard's Manual of Operative Dentistry

Ninth edition

Avijit Banerjee

Senior Lecturer/Honorary Consultant, Restorative Dentistry
King's College London Dental Institute at Guy's, King's College and St Thomas' Hospitals,
KCL, London, UK
and
Visiting Professor, Restorative Dentistry, Oman Dental College, Oman

Timothy F Watson

Professor of Biomaterials and Restorative Dentistry/Honorary Consultant, Restorative Dentistry
King's College London Dental Institute at Guy's, King's College and St Thomas' Hospitals,
KCL, London, UK

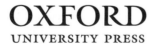

OXFORD
UNIVERSITY PRESS

OXFORD

UNIVERSITY PRESS

Great Clarendon Street, Oxford OX2 6DP

Oxford University Press is a department of the University of Oxford.
It furthers the University's objective of excellence in research, scholarship,
and education by publishing worldwide in

Oxford New York

Auckland Cape Town Dar es Salaam Hong Kong Karachi
Kuala Lumpur Madrid Melbourne Mexico City Nairobi
New Delhi Shanghai Taipei Toronto

With offices in

Argentina Austria Brazil Chile Czech Republic France Greece
Guatemala Hungary Italy Japan Poland Portugal Singapore
South Korea Switzerland Thailand Turkey Ukraine Vietnam

Oxford is a registered trade mark of Oxford University Press
in the UK and in certain other countries

Published in the United States
by Oxford University Press Inc., New York

British Library Cataloguing in Publication Data
Data available

Library of Congress Cataloging in Publication Data
Data available

Typeset by TNQ, India
Printed and bound in UK by
Bell & Bain Ltd., Glasgow

ISBN 978-0-19-957915-0

3 5 7 9 10 8 6 4

Foreword

It is a great pleasure and honour to prepare the Foreword for the ninth edition of *Pickard's Manual of Operative Dentistry (Pickard)*, one of the most highly regarded and widely used books in dentistry.

Nothing endures more than change, and with change comes new concepts, processes, and goals to be adopted. Operative dentistry has undergone tremendous change in recent years, with new understanding of dental diseases, developments in diagnostic technologies, novel approaches to prevention, a shift to minimally interventive techniques, facilitated by advances in dental adhesives and restorative systems, and new thinking in respect to the maintenance and repair of restored teeth. It is no surprise, therefore, that large elements of *Pickard* have had to be re-prepared and added to in the production of this ninth edition, which has both a new look and a new author.

As would be expected of a book of the standing of *Pickard*, the new edition is not only comprehensive, authoritative, and evidence-based, it is well produced, attractively illustrated, and user friendly, whether read cover to cover or dipped into for information in respect of specific aspects of operative dentistry. To achieve these qualities in a book, covering a major element of the clinical practice of dentistry, is no mean feat. As a consequence, the authors of this new, timely edition of *Pickard* are to be congratulated on a job well done, in particular, given the ways in which the text takes account of subtle differences in approach within and between the many countries of the world in which the book will undoubtedly have great appeal.

With the publication and wide-ranging use of this excellent new edition of *Pickard*, it is to be hoped that the shift to minimally invasive dentistry, including the adoption of biological rather than mechanistic approaches to the management of caries, will be all the more rapid. Paraphrasing GV Black, the day has surely arrived when the practice of operative dentistry is more about prevention and the preservation of tooth tissues than traumatic reparative dentistry. In this way, it is anticipated that this new, ninth edition of *Pickard* may come to be viewed as a historic watershed between the traditional and modern art and science of operative dentistry.

I unreservedly recommend this book to all members of the dental team, in particular, existing practitioners, dental therapists, and other dental care professionals, students, and teachers alike. It is to be hoped that the knowledge and principles eloquently discussed and described in this book will be widely and effectively applied in the interests of future generations of patients, let alone the modernization of the clinical practice of operative dentistry. For students of operative dentistry at all levels and all other oral healthcare students seeking state of the art knowledge and understanding in respect of modern restorative dentistry, do not look back; use this book as the foundation for your future clinical practice. For existing practitioners, therapists, and teachers, put the past behind you and embrace 21st-century operative dentistry. Enjoy and use this excellent new edition of *Pickard* to the best possible advantage.

Nairn Wilson CBE DSc (*hc*) FDS FKC

Preface to the ninth edition

It is nearly 50 years since the first edition of this book was published. The continuing philosophy underpinning operative dentistry as initially proposed by Professor Pickard and continued under the authorship of Professors Kidd and Smith is as valid now as it was in 1962. This philosophy has several strands, which are all inter-related.

- Dentists and dental care professionals primarily look after people with dental problems – not just mouths or teeth.

- An understanding of the disease processes is fundamental to their management.

- The diseases should be managed – not just treated.

- Prevention, patient motivation, and tailoring of dental care to their carefully assessed requirements is the keystone of management.

- When active treatment is needed, the choice of materials and techniques should be based on a thorough understanding of them and the advantages and disadvantages of the alternatives.

- Once operative intervention is called for, science, technology, and good, old-fashioned craft skills should deliver a standard of care with which the patient will be happy and the operator proud. However, although the practical and theoretical requirements should be apparent from reading this book, technical skills will only go so far: we still require excellent clinical teachers to inspire students and pass on their full knowledge of patient care. Practice *can* make perfect and operative dentistry is not a skill that is picked up overnight!

Operative dentistry is a continuously evolving discipline, and prefaces to previous editions have highlighted some of these changes. As an example, there is now no question that tooth-coloured restorative materials can be used in most operative treatments. This is not to say that the alternatives such as amalgam and gold are no longer effective or indicated, but that with careful use, modern materials are just as capable of producing durable and acceptable restorations. Indeed, the environmental issues surrounding amalgam will probably cause its demise rather than any direct patient-related factors. For this reason, the trend started in the seventh and eighth editions of this book has been continued with further downplaying of its clinical application.

Pickard is a 'Manual of Operative Dentistry': the intention is that this book contains the material a dental student or dental care professional needs to know (excluding endodontic and periodontal treatment) up to the point that laboratory-made restorations become necessary. In other words, students can learn to provide disease management and long-term stabilization, including permanent intra-coronal restorations and cores for crowns. In this edition, examples of practical techniques available have increased, especially attempting to produce clear descriptions of the implications of the interactions between restorative materials and tooth tissue. This cannot be achieved without increasing some of the theoretical background to the practice of operative dentistry, especially in underpinning disciplines such as dental histology, cariology, and dental materials science. As a result, we hope that this edition will be as applicable to the final year dental/dental care professional student (and graduate) as one about to embark on their first operative clinical skills course. In response to feedback from undergraduates and clinical teachers, we have changed the book's format. It should be easier to extract information from the text as there are many more flowcharts, tables, heavily captioned and illustrated technique photographs, and 'less words'. Almost uniquely, this textbook has got smaller with this new edition! Self-testing has also been introduced in each section, which may not be exhaustive but goes some way to challenge the reader to think about the clinical application of what they have just read.

Teachers of operative dentistry will recognize much in this book that has survived from previous editions. Without Bernard Smith and Edwina Kidd keeping this textbook at the forefront of the teaching in operative dentistry over the last 20 years, we would not have had the solid foundations on which to build this evolving textbook, capable of reflecting the current state of play in our discipline. We sincerely thank them for their support and encouragement over the years.

We wish to thank our many colleagues who have allowed us to use their illustrations. They are acknowledged in the captions to the relevant figures together with a source of the original publication where applicable.

AB

TFW

August 2010

Contents

1

Dental hard tissue pathologies, aetiology, and their clinical manifestations

Chapter contents

1.1 Introduction: why practise operative dentistry?

Technically, operative dentistry is that aspect of restorative dentistry which directly repairs and/or restores damaged and defective teeth in order to maintain structure, function, and aesthetics. The damage or defects can be caused by one or more of the following:

- Caries
- Toothwear
- Trauma
- Developmental conditions.

The principles of operative dentistry must also include methods of detection, diagnosis, and control/prevention of the above conditions, as care planning involves the whole patient, not just restoring damaged or defective teeth in isolation. The following sections will provide an overview of these four conditions with respect to their aetiology, histopathology, and microbiology where relevant. An attempt will be made to relate these features to the clinical manifestations of each condition, namely carious lesions and toothwear lesions.

1.2 Dental caries

1.2.1 Definition

Dental caries is a reversible (in its earliest stages), progressive disease of the dental hard tissues, instigated by the action of bacteria upon fermentable carbohydrates in the plaque biofilm on tooth surfaces, leading to acid demineralization and ultimately proteolytic destruction of the organic component of the dental tissues.

1.2.2 Terminology

Primary caries is the process and lesion occurring on a previously sound tooth surface.

Root caries is primary caries on an exposed root surface (usually after gingival recession has occurred), often penetrating more easily into the exposed dentine. The pathological process for both primary and root caries is the same (see Figures 1.1, 1.2).

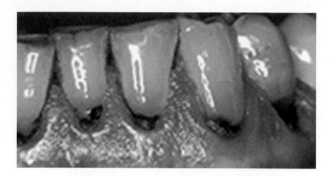

Figure 1.1 Slowly progressing root surface lesions with dark, leathery dentine surfaces and some plaque deposits. This is the mouth of a 70-year-old patient with a dry mouth (xerostomia, 2° Sjögren's syndrome) and rheumatoid arthritis, making oral hygiene difficult due to impaired toothbrush manipulation and painful mucosae.

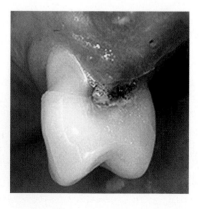

Figure 1.2 An active root caries lesion with overlying plaque deposit in an area of stagnation alongside the margins of a partial denture. The buccal cervical abrasion cavity has been caused by excessive toothbrushing.

Recurrent (secondary) caries is primary caries occurring at the margin of a restoration. The aetiology is the same – metabolic activity in the plaque biofilm. *Residual caries* is an older term designating that portion of the caries-affected, demineralized tissue left behind in a cavity that is then restored (see later).

1.2.3 Caries: the process and the lesion

The carious process

The carious process is the metabolic activity in the plaque biofilm resident on the tooth surface. This biofilm begins to form just a few minutes after the tooth surface has been brushed, and is initially adsorbed as the acquired pellicle containing salivary proteins and glycoproteins. With time, oral bacteria colonize the biofilm closely associated with bacterial extracellular polysaccharides and salivary proteins. With time, the increased density of the developing biofilm, changing bacterial population, pH, and oxygen tension all combine to create a cariogenic environment on the tooth surface. This ubiquitous, natural, metabolic process cannot be *prevented*. However, disease progression can be *controlled* so that a clinically visible enamel lesion never forms. The de- and remineralization metabolic processes can be modified particularly by regular disturbance of the biofilm with a toothbrush and fluoride toothpaste. If the biofilm is partially or totally removed, mineral loss may be stopped or even reversed towards mineral gain (in very early lesions). The fluoride in toothpaste delays lesion progression by inhibiting demineralization and encouraging remineralization.

The carious lesion

The carious lesion forms as a direct consequence of the metabolic activity in the biofilm on the tooth surface, i.e. the carious process. If factors tip the de-/remineralization balance towards demineralization (plaque, diet, and time), the stages of progressive lesion formation leading to cavitation can be clinically detected and dealt with accordingly.

1.2.4 Aetiology of the caries process

Occurring ubiquitously in the plaque biofilm, the main factors that interplay in the aetiology of the carious process are:

- *Bacteria*: with colonization within the plaque biofilm, several hundred different species exist within a complex ecology, dependent on the age and relative stagnancy of the plaque on the tooth surface. *Streptococcus mutans*, classically thought to be the primary causative bacterial species, has recently been considered to have more of an associative role in the caries process and may act as a microbiological marker for caries. *Lactobacillus* and *bifidobacteria* species have been shown to be significant in the caries process and it is likely that species interaction within the biofilm will instigate and allow the carious lesion to progress.

- *Susceptible tooth surfaces (see Chapter 2)*: Carious lesions occur on tooth surfaces that have accumulated plaque, stagnating for a prolonged period of time, which may include:
  - The depths of pits and fissures on posterior occlusal/buccal surfaces of those teeth which a patient cannot clean effectively with a toothbrush. These areas on newly erupting molars are particularly susceptible to carious attack.
  - Approximal surfaces (mesial and distal) *cervical* to the contact points of adjacent teeth (where patients may not floss regularly/at all). These surfaces of particularly imbricated (crowded) teeth can be more susceptible due to the lack of access for oral hygiene aids.
  - Smooth surfaces adjacent to the gingival margin (again an area that patients may often miss with their toothbrush).
  - The ledged/overhanging/defective margins of restorations (a plaque trap often inaccessible to a toothbrush or floss) (see Figure 1.3).

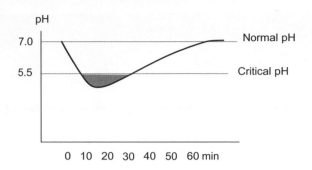

Figure 1.4 The Stephan curve, showing the changes in plaque pH over time after an oral glucose rinse at time 0 min. The critical pH of enamel is that below which the hydroxyapatite crystals begin to dissociate into ions. The grey-shaded portion of the graph indicates the 20-min period in which the tooth surface is under threat of mineral loss. In dentine, the critical pH of mineral is 6.2.

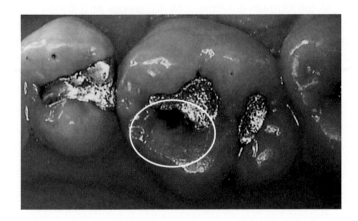

Figure 1.3 Caries at the margin of the failed amalgam restoration (white circle) on the occlusal surface of UL6 (see Chapter 2 for a description of tooth notation).

- *Fermentable carbohydrates*: the plaque bacteria are capable of metabolizing certain dietary carbohydrates (including sucrose and glucose) producing various organic acids (lactic, acetic, propionic acids) at the tooth surface causing plaque pH to fall within one to three minutes and initiating demineralization if the pH drops to below 5.5 (critical pH). The pH can take up to 60 minutes to climb back to normal, aided by the buffering capacity of saliva (pH 7.0; see Figure 1.4). This demineralization/remineralization cycle occurs continuously at any tooth surface, all the time.
- *Time*: even though the drop in pH commences rapidly, sufficient time is required for the plaque biofilm to produce a *net* mineral loss equating to hard tissue damage at the tooth surface.

The four above direct causes can be affected/modified by several other indirect patient factors to ultimately affect the disease pattern experienced by each individual patient. These determinants include the patient's:

- Income (the cost of dental care)
- Knowledge about their own oral health

- Attitudes to healthcare
- Social class
- Behaviour
- Education.

These factors can be assessed during history taking and oral examination (Chapter 2) and help form the basis of determining the individual's own risk of developing caries – the caries risk assessment (Chapter 3).

1.2.5 Speed and severity of the carious process

The carious process in the normal oral environment will take several weeks to become clinically detectable as lesions with signs and symptoms. This is because the overall process, with its continuously fluctuating metabolic balance at the ionic level, is relatively slow and can be moderated by oral hygiene techniques, dietary modification, and the use of fluoride. The presence of saliva, with its capacity to buffer plaque acids and remove food debris and lubricate tooth surfaces also helps.

Rampant caries However, clinical scenarios exist where the process is accelerated and many lesions form rapidly, often involving surfaces of teeth ordinarily relatively caries-free – rampant caries. This classically affects the primary dentition (nursing/bottle caries; see Figure 1.5), teenagers, or young adults with a highly cariogenic diet (frequent sugar episodes; see Figure 1.6) and/or addicted to recreational drugs, or in adult patients with a dry mouth (xerostomia). Radiation in the region of the salivary glands, used in the treatment of an orofacial malignant growth, and Sjögren's syndrome, an autoimmune condition which may involve the salivary glands, are the most common causes of severe xerostomia. In addition, a large number of therapeutic drugs, such as antidepressants, tranquillizers, antihypertensives, and diuretics can retard salivary flow.

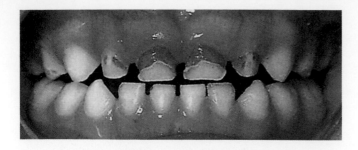

Figure 1.5 Rampant caries affecting deciduous anterior teeth.

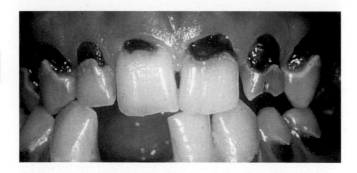

Figure 1.6 Rampant caries in an adult patient with cavities affecting sites not normally associated with caries due to their accessibility for adequate oral hygiene.

Arrested caries In distinct contrast to rampant caries, the term arrested caries describes lesions which have stopped progressing and are inactive. It is seen when the oral environment has changed from conditions predisposing to caries to conditions that tend to slow lesion progression. These lesions often have a dark, hard, shiny exposed dentine surface (see Figure 1.7).

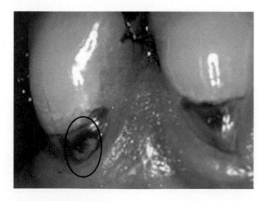

Figure 1.7 A hard, shiny and stained arrested root surface lesion on the buccal cervical aspect of the canine. Plaque is evident on a portion of a similar lesion on the first premolar indicating that this area is likely to be active (black circle).

1.2.6 The carious lesion

Having summarized the caries process as an ongoing, metabolic de-/remineralization balance occurring at the interface between the plaque biofilm and the tooth surface, it is important to understand that the carious lesion is a progressive alteration and destruction of the hard tissues (mineral and organic matrix) from the enamel surface through to the pulp. While the lesion is still within enamel, it can be arrested and possibly reversed in its earliest stages. Once into dentine, the process can be arrested but if proteolytic destruction of the organic collagen matrix has occurred, this cannot be histologically reversed. This section will take the reader through key features of the histological and clinical development of a lesion from its earliest enamel stages through to cavitation into the pulp.

An understanding of the basic histological features of healthy enamel and dentine is a prerequisite to appreciating the changes that occur within the lesion and an outline of these is presented in Table 6.1, Chapter 6. Further information can be gathered from aids offered in the Appendix. The relationship between lesion histology and clinical appearance has been used in a caries detection and assessment system outlined and discussed in Chapter 2 (Table 2.3).

Within enamel

Plaque-acid demineralization causes porosities to form within the prism structure, initially beneath the outer surface of enamel: this is subsurface demineralization. The developing pore volumes through the depth of the enamel lesion, caused by a longer exposure to reduced pH, have been measured using polarized light microscopy (outermost

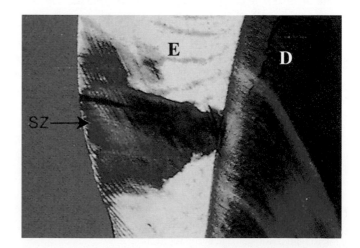

Figure 1.8 Longitudinal ground section through a carious lesion on a smooth surface (polarized light and water; E, enamel; D, dentine). The enamel lesion is shaped as an inverted cone, widest at the tooth surface, narrowing towards the enamel–dentine junction, with a relatively intact surface zone (SZ).

surface zone (<1% pore volume), body (5–25%), dark (2–4%) and innermost translucent zone (1%); see Figure 1.8).

The existence of the enamel lesion surface zone may be due to increased extrinsic fluoride ion deposition in this area or as a consequence of remineralization metabolism of the biofilm on the tooth surface. It is essential that this intact surface is not iatrogenically cavitated (that is, a hole created by a dentist sticking a sharp dental probe into the lesion surface) as it has the potential to heal if the biofilm can be regularly and effectively removed, and remineralizing solutions and/or toothpastes containing higher concentrations of calcium and phosphate ions, are used.

Histologically, smooth surface lesions have a cross-sectional shape of an inverted cone (widest superficially, apex towards the enamel–dentine junction (EDJ); see Figure 1.12). Fissure lesions take the form of two adjacent smooth surface lesions (see Figure 1.9).

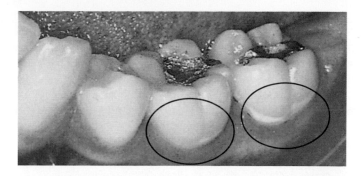

Figure 1.10 Early white spot enamel lesions on the cervical-gingival margins of both mandibular left molars (circled).

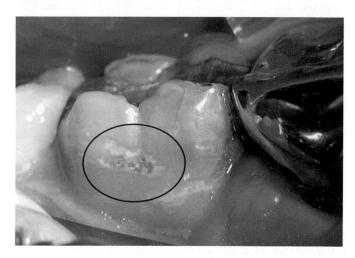

Figure 1.11 Active white spot enamel lesion on the mid-buccal of LL7 (circled). This more developed lesion has a rough surface, acting as a plaque trap.

Q1.11: What features of this lesion will help the dentist conclude that it is active, how might these be detected, and how might the patient be managed?

If plaque is removed, lesions can arrest and porosities can be eliminated due to abrasive toothwear, resulting in the hard, smooth, shiny surfaces of arrested lesions. Porosities may also be filled with deposited mineral and dietary molecules causing staining (e.g. tannins), which may be trapped within the mineral lattice. This creates an arrested, brown spot lesion (BSL) with a hard, shiny overlying smooth surface.

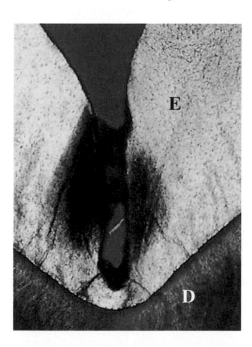

Figure 1.9 A longitudinal ground section (polarized light with water) through an occlusal fissure showing an enamel lesion forming on the two adjacent walls of the fissure (dark regions; E, enamel; D, dentine).

Q1.9: How might this scenario be managed in a high caries risk patient?

Clinical manifestations the active white spot lesion (WSL) is initially smooth, frosty white/opaque, and non-cavitated (see Figure 1.10). This can be detected more easily if the tooth surface is air-dried for a few seconds using a 3-1 air/water syringe. As the lesion develops over time, it becomes somewhat chalky, eventually becoming roughened or micro-cavitated (detected by gently running a blunt probe across the lesion surface). This can encourage further plaque deposition (see Figure 1.11). There are no symptoms at this stage, but reactions in the dentine–pulp complex may be mediated by cytokines and bacterial breakdown products within the dentine matrix and tubules (see later).

The EDJ or the amelo–dentinal junction (ADJ)

Histologically, the carious process may reach dentine before clinical cavitation is detectable (a closed lesion: mICDAS score 2, see Chapter 2). Defence reactions in the dentine–pulp complex are stimulated at this stage with evidence of translucent dentine at the lesion boundary and tertiary dentine deposition at the dentine–pulp interface beneath the advancing lesion (see later). Again, symptoms are unlikely at this stage of lesion development.

The lesion extends in dentine, immediately subjacent to the EDJ (see Figure 1.12), its extension coinciding with the spread of the enamel lesion at the surface of the tooth, which in turn is dependent on the extent of the plaque biofilm at the tooth surface. Relative hypomineralization in this zone of mantle dentine, greater side-branching of dentine tubules or defects within the enamel/dentine interface may also contribute to this spread.

The lesion can then penetrate along the dentine tubules towards the pulp.

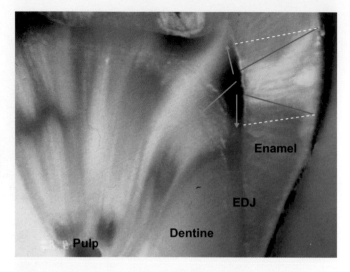

Figure 1.12 A mesiodistal section through a carious tooth highlighting an approximal lesion. The red lines outline the 'inverted cone' cross-sectional histological shape of the enamel lesion and the blue lines the direction of spread of the lesion having crossed the enamel–dentine junction (EDJ) into dentine. The white dotted lines show how the extent of the spread of the dentine lesion subjacent to the EDJ is associated with the same lateral extent of the enamel lesion on the tooth surface, both governed by the presence of the plaque biofilm at the tooth surface.

Within dentine

Once the lesion has spread histologically approximately into the middle third of dentine, it is often clinically cavitated (open) on both occlusal and smooth surfaces with plaque now able to accumulate on the exposed dentine surface. The spread of the lesion will undermine the overlying enamel, with an associated grey shadow/opacity, which becomes brittle and prone to fracture under occlusal loading. This may need to be removed during cavity preparation (Chapter 7).

The patient may experience initial symptoms of acute pulpitis – a poorly localized sharp pain of a few seconds duration stimulated by hot, cold, or sweet (Chapter 3). The components of carious dentine to be considered are the mineral, collagen, bacterial penetration and tubule structure. Both degenerative and reparative processes act on these simultaneously in different parts of the lesion. The histological changes of the carious dentine biomass through its depth (from EDJ to pulp) are described below, but note that these descriptive zones are not separate biological entities, but blend into one another without clear boundaries (see Figure 1.13).

- *Caries-infected dentine* (zone 1, Figure 1.13): the outermost, superficial, irreparable, necrotic zone of destruction often clinically distinguished as a dark brown, soft, wet, 'mushy' layer.
  - Mineral component has dissolved away due to acid attack
  - Collagenous matrix has been denatured (irreparable damage) by proteolytic enzymes from bacteria and intrinsic to the dentine itself (the zinc-dependent matrix metalloproteinases (MMPs)), activated by bacterial acids produced during the carious process
  - Bacterial load in this zone is very high
  - Dentine tubular structure is destroyed.
- This zone should be clinically removed when preparing a cavity as it is necrotic, cannot be repaired, and provides a poor quality bonding substrate for adhesive materials to achieve an adequate seal.
- *Caries-affected dentine* (zones 2, 3, 4 combined together; Figure 1.13): the inner layer of carious dentine which can be repaired by the dentine–pulp complex, often distinguished as paler brown, harder, 'sticky and scratchy' dentine (to a sharp probe, but not used over the pulpal floor of the cavity).
  - Mineral dissolution still occurs but to a lesser extent than infected dentine, as the pH gradually rises towards the advancing front of the lesion
  - Collagen is still damaged by proteolysis but to a lesser extent so permitting dentine repair, as the proteinaceous scaffold for mineral crystal deposition persists
  - Bacterial load lessens but there are still bacteria present
  - Dentine tubular structure returns gradually within the depths of this zone.
- The deepest layer of caries-affected dentine (zone 4, Figure 1.13) can be described as hypermineralized translucent dentine (due to its glassy appearance in cross-section), one of several reparative reactions of the dentine–pulp complex to the carious process (see later). As can be seen in Figures 1.12 and 1.13, the lesion in dentine often has a dark brown discoloration within the caries-infected zone, which then gradually pales through the depth of the lesion, towards the pulp. The aetiology of the colour changes is not clear but a biochemical reaction between proteins and carbohydrates in a moist, acidic biological environment, the *Maillard reaction*, may play a part. Not all lesions are uniformly dark brown; some rapidly advancing lesions may have a pale discoloration within the caries-infected zone and there is no direct link between the colour of dentine and the bacteria present within these zones.

1.2.7 Carious pulp exposure

If the carious process cannot be modified and the lesion is not treated in time with appropriate excavation and restoration within the dentine, then the advancing front of the lesion approaches the dentine–pulp boundary and bacteria/toxins will penetrate the pulpal tissues causing an acute inflammatory response. Depending on the time scale over which this has happened, an initial acute pulpitic response (poorly localized short, sharp pain on hot, cold or sweet stimuli) will evolve into a more chronic response, changing symptoms towards a dull, prolonged ache that may last several minutes and is spontaneous and

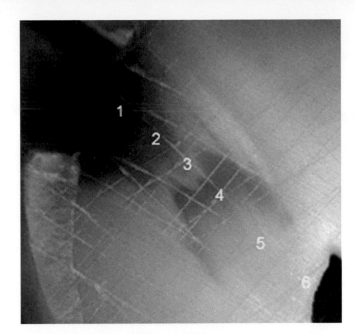

Figure 1.13 A mesiodistal section through an approximal lesion showing a cavity in the enamel and the histological colour changes through the dentine lesion (1, caries-infected dentine; 2, 3, and 4, caries-affected dentine; 4, translucent dentine; 5, 6, sound dentine). The surface scratches were placed to act as reference markers during microscopic analysis of the sample.

Q1.13: What causes the colour change in dentine caries?

non-specific in origin (Chapter 3). The cavity will probably have enlarged due to the undermined enamel having been broken away (including marginal ridges of proximal lesions) and will be noticeable to the patient as 'a hole in the tooth'.

If the pulp chamber is breached by the lesion, a *carious exposure* may be created when excavating very deep caries, and the exposed pulpal tissue will bleed uncontrollably for several minutes before cotton wool pledgets can achieve haemostasis. In most cases of a carious pulpal exposure, root canal treatment is the management option of choice (as long as the tooth is restorable with a worthwhile prognosis), but this will depend on the size of the exposure, the age of the patient (a young, well-vascularized pulp may have a better prognosis) and the severity of the carious process within the depth of the lesion (Chapter 5). In rare cases, on late presentation, the pulpal soft tissues undergo a hyperplastic cellular reaction and appear to herniate through the exposure, into the cavity.

1.2.8 Dentine–pulp complex reparative reactions

Dentine is a vital tissue containing the cytoplasmic extensions of odontoblasts and must be considered together with the pulp since the two tissues are so intimately connected. The dentine–pulp complex, like any other vital tissue in the body, is capable of defending itself. The state of the tissue at any time will depend on the balance between the attacking forces and the defence reactions. The defence reactions include deposition of *translucent dentine*, *tertiary dentine*, and *pulpal inflammation*.

Translucent dentine

Sometimes referred to as 'sclerotic' dentine, this glassy zone of dentine (zone 4, Figure 1.13) is caused by tubular infill with plate-like Whitlockite mineral crystals (β-octocalciumphosphate) at the advancing front of the lesion in an attempt to wall-off the advancing lesion. Its appearance is due to the parity of refractive indices of intertubular and intratubular mineral, so allowing light to pass through the sectioned boundaries.

The Whitlockite deposits originate from a combination of a physico-chemical re-precipitation of calcium and phosphate ions diffusing towards the increasing pH environment of the lesion's deepest advancing front and also possibly a vital process of new and rapid mineral deposition from the pulp via the odontoblasts. Even though hypermineralized, this zone of translucent dentine is softer than its deeper, sound counterpart due to the weaker crystalline orientation of Whitlockite than conventional hydroxyapatite crystals within the tubules (similar to stacking dinner plates flat – too tall a stack and they topple over!) (see Figure 1.14).

Tertiary (reactionary/reparative/irritation/atubular) dentine

This is the dentine that is laid down at the dentine–pulp border in response to a noxious stimulus, e.g. caries or those causing toothwear, in an attempt to wall off and distance the pulp from the advancing noxious stimuli (see Figure 1.15). It may resemble secondary dentine histologically, but has an irregular tubular or atubular structure, depending on the speed of its creation. Reactionary dentine is deposited as a result of a mild irritant where original odontoblasts survive and are metabolically upregulated. Reparative dentine is deposited in response to a stronger irritant which compromises the vitality of the original odontoblasts. Progenitor cells from the subodontoblastic layer then differentiate and are upregulated to produce an atubular defence reaction.

Pulp inflammation

This is the fundamental response of all vascular connective tissues to injury. Inflammation of the pulp (pulpitis) may, as in any other tissue, be acute or chronic. In a slowly progressing carious lesion, toxins reaching the pulp may provoke chronic inflammation. However, once the organisms actually reach the pulp (a carious exposure), acute inflammation may supervene. Inflammatory reactions have vascular and cellular components. In chronic inflammation the cellular components predominate and there may be increased collagen production, leading to fibrosis but without immediately endangering the vitality of the tooth. However, in acute inflammation the vascular changes predominate.

Infection is the most common cause of pulpal inflammation and caries is the most common microbial source. Dentine caries will result in pulpal inflammation and chronic inflammatory cells (macrophages, lymphocytes, and plasma cells) will infiltrate the pulp near the odonto-

1

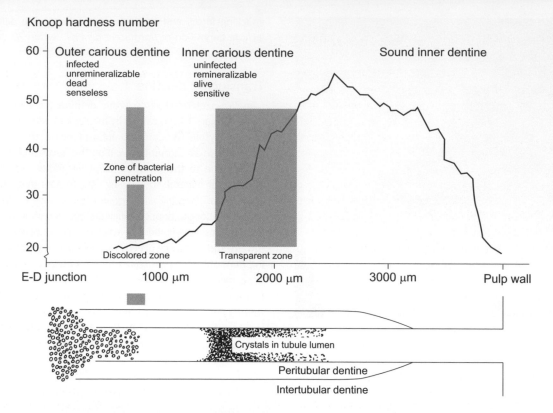

Figure 1.14 labels (within chart):

Knoop hardness number

Outer carious dentine
infected
unremineralizable
dead
senseless

Inner carious dentine
uninfected
remineralizable
alive
sensitive

Sound inner dentine

Zone of bacterial penetration

Discolored zone

Transparent zone

E-D junction   1000 μm   2000 μm   3000 μm   Pulp wall

Crystals in tubule lumen

Peritubular dentine

Intertubular dentine

Figure 1.14 Chart showing the changes in hardness of carious dentine (y-axis) from the enamel–dentine junction (EDJ) towards the pulp (x-axis) and relating this to the histological changes that occur through the dentine lesion. The transparent zone (synonymous with the translucent zone) is softer than the deeper, less mineralized, sound dentine. The diagram equates the bacterial content and mineral deposition within the tubule lumen through the progressive zones of carious dentine. (From Ogawa *et al.* (1983), taken from Fejerskov and Kidd (2008) *Dental caries – the disease and its clinical management*, Chichester: Wiley.)

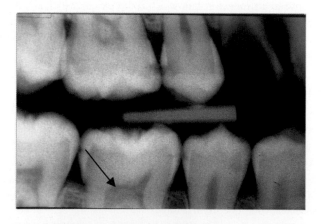

Figure 1.15 Right bitewing radiograph of a patient with high caries rate and multiple lesions. Note the dentine–pulp complex reparative response of LR6 to the distal dentine lesion – the distal pulp horn has been obliterated by deposits of tertiary dentine (arrow).

Q1.15: How many other carious lesions can you detect?

blast layer. Indeed, this infiltration may even be seen in response to initial enamel caries. This chronic inflammatory reaction is mainly due to the movement of bacterial toxins through the dentinal tubules. Secretory immunoglobulins travel in the dentinal fluid up the remaining patent tubules. With increasing carious involvement of enamel and dentine, the area of chronic inflammation increases in size but it is believed to remain localized until pulp exposure. Bacteria may enter the pulp with polymorphonuclear leucocytes predominating and acute inflammation can supervene, spread throughout the pulp and result in pulpal necrosis.

1.3 Toothwear ('tooth surface loss')

Toothwear is the irreversible surface loss of dental hard tissues caused by factors other than caries or trauma. Toothwear (TW) can be physiological, occurring slowly, naturally throughout life, or pathological, occurring at a much faster rate, usually caused by combinations of erosion, attrition, abrasion, and perhaps abfraction (Table 1.1).

Erosion is the irreversible loss of dental hard tissues by a chemical process (acid attack) not involving bacteria. It is often the common denominator in the multifactorial aetiology of toothwear. Sources of acid can either be intrinsic (stomach acid regurgitation) or extrinsic (dietary, environmental). Involuntary gastro-oesophageal reflux disease (GORD) is a common cause of intrinsic stomach acids entering the oral cavity on a regular basis and occurs primarily due to transient relaxation or incompetence of the lower oesophageal sphincter. Certain factors in combination often predispose to GORD, and these factors may include:

- Diet – fatty, spicy foods consumed in large quantities especially late at night
- Alcohol
- Certain medications, e.g. diazepam
- Causes of increased gastric pressure including obesity, pregnancy, posture (lying down increases pressure on the sphincter) and even excessive exercise
- Gastro-oesophageal reflux predisposes to further GORD symptoms
- Neuromuscular conditions.

Treatment for GORD will depend on the aetiology. As well as conservative management involving modifying diet, lifestyle and the use of chewing gum, stomach acids can be neutralized using conventional antacids (e.g. Gaviscon) or their production limited with oral medications including proton pump inhibitors (e.g. omeprazole (Losec)) or H_2 antagonists (e.g. cimetidine). Surgical procedures can

Table 1.1 Toothwear: common aetiology, features and simple classification

Aetiological factors		Comments
Erosion	Intrinsic, regurgitation (GORD, vomiting)	Most common cause of erosion; affects palatal surfaces maxillary anteriors, occlusal/buccal surfaces of lower molars. Stomach hydrochloric acid originates from: <ul><li>Involuntary GORD</li><li>Involuntary/voluntary vomiting.</li></ul>
	Extrinsic, dietary	Affects labial surfaces of maxillary anteriors. ↓ pH due to excess acidic food/drink intake: <ul><li>Citrus fruit and fruit juices</li><li>Pickles, vinegar-containing foodstuffs</li><li>Carbonated drinks (including diet/health drinks)</li><li>Some mouthwashes have a low pH.</li></ul> Drinking habits: through straw and frothing around mouth. Acids include citric, carbonic, acetic, hydrochloric, phosphoric acids. Often associated with a healthy lifestyle – patient understanding required to modify erosive potential of the diet.
	Extrinsic, environmental	Labial surfaces of maxillary anteriors/pitting. Rare nowadays due to stringent health and safety regulations in the workplace. Historically industrial processes where acid was vaporized and inhaled (battery manufacturers, tanning factories).
Attrition		TW caused by occlusal tooth–tooth contact; occlusal facets match with opposing teeth; usually in combination with erosion. Often caused by grinding/parafunctional habits.
Abrasion		TW caused by tooth–non-tooth contact; hard toothbrushing with coarse toothpastes, dish-/V-shaped, smooth cervical lesions; incisal wear/grooves from long-term habitual behaviour, e.g. pipe smokers, milliners holding pins between their teeth, builders holding nails, etc.
Abfraction (contentious)		Cervical V-shaped enamel–dentine TW lesions with no history of abrasion. Aetiology not clear, but masticatory stresses may concentrate at cervical margins of teeth and perhaps open up pre-existing cracks/weaknesses in the tooth.

GORD, gastro-oesophageal reflux disease.

be carried out to repair physical damage to the gastro-oesophageal system. Once this is done, any dental damage can be repaired. The patient's dentist may often be the first to notice the problem through the dental manifestations and appropriate referral to medical colleagues may be required.

Intrinsic acids can also enter the oral cavity through voluntary or involuntary vomiting, causes of which include:

● Psychosomatic:

– Eating disorders:

» Bulimia nervosa (affects 1–2% adolescent population; F:M ratio, 10:1)

» Anorexia nervosa (affects 0.1–1% of the teenage population; F:M ratio, 10:1)

– Rumination (voluntary regurgitation followed by re-digestion of stomach contents)

– Stress-induced psychogenic vomiting

● Metabolic/endocrine:

– pregnancy

● Gastro-intestinal disorders:

– Peptic ulcer/gastritis

– Hiatus hernia

– Achalasia – a condition associated with a narrowed lower oesophageal sphincter and reduced oesophageal motility leading to stagnation and fermentation of ingested food within the oesophagus and concomitant regurgitation

– Cerebral palsy

● Drug induced:

– Primary – cytotoxics

– Secondary – gastric irritation, alcohol, aspirin, and other non-steroidal anti-inflammatory medications.

Again, in the above cases, the initial cause of the vomiting must be found out from the patient's history and examination and the cause itself treated first before restoring any damaged dentition (see Chapter 2), with close cooperation with the patient's medical practitioner.

The aetiology and features of abrasion and attrition have been outlined in Table 1.1. Erosion is often a contributory factor in the overall pattern of clinical toothwear. Acid-softened tooth surfaces are more susceptible to long-term 'wear' forces from opposing teeth (attrition) or other external influences (abrasion). Clinical examples of these are shown in Chapter 2.

1.4 Dental trauma

While caries and toothwear are diseases of relatively slow onset, traumatic injuries are acquired suddenly, and when these involve the hard dental tissues and the pulp they usually require immediate operative management to stabilize the condition, provide pain relief and restore function and appearance if possible. Trauma to the mouth can produce any combination of the following local injuries:

● Lacerations to the lips, tongue, buccal and gingival tissue

● Alveolar fractures, so that a number of teeth become mobile within a block of bone

● Complete or partial subluxation of a tooth

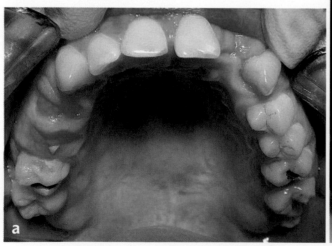
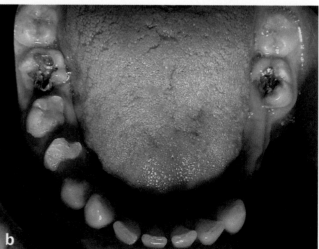

Figure 1.16a, b Maxillary and mandibular occlusal views of a patient having sustained multiple facial blows in a fight. Note the decoronated UR45 and large enamel and dentine fractures sustained on UR6, UL7, LR4,5,6, and LL6. UL2 and LL45 were avulsed in the incident.

Q1.16: What might have been the presenting dental complaints for the above patient?

- Root fracture
- Damage to the apical blood vessels without fracture
- Fracture of the crown of the tooth involving enamel alone, enamel and dentine, or exposure of the pulp (see Figure 2.25, Chapter 2).

1.4.1 Aetiology

Trauma is commonly caused by the following:

- Falls
- Sports/athletics injuries
- Blows from heavy objects
- Fights
- Car/bicycle accidents
- Injuries sustained during convulsive seizures (e.g. epilepsy)
- Battered child syndrome (the most difficult and yet the most important to diagnose).

Detection and management will be discussed in subsequent chapters. Examples of dental trauma can be seen in Figures 1.16 and 1.17.

In some cases, untreated traumatic injury can lead to the development of long-term pathology (see Figure 1.17).

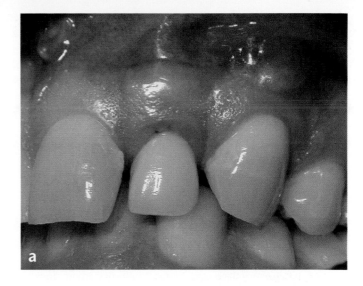

Figure 1.17 (**a**) A fit and well young adult has sustained an accidental blow to the teeth in the UL123 area several months earlier.

Q1.17a: Can you detect any abnormal clinical findings from the above picture (clue – check the mucosae)?

1

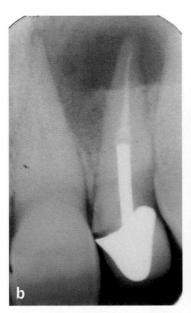
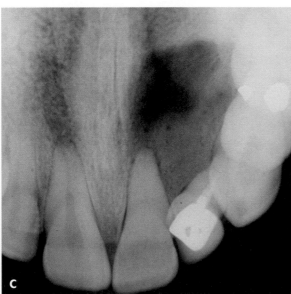
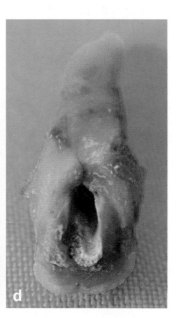

Figure 1.17 (**b**) Periapical and (**c**) upper standard occlusal (USO) radiographs of the UL123 shown in (**a**). Note the large well-demarcated pathological radiolucency originating from the root apex of the fractured and displaced root, post-core and crown complex in the UL2. The lesion is tracking in the overlying mucosa to the swelling visible in (**a**). (**d**) The extracted UL2 root with the post-core and crown removed showing the crack sustained from the impact.

Q1.17c: What other findings are evident from the USO?

1.5 Developmental defects

Teeth do not always develop normally and there are a number of defects in tooth structure or shape which occur during development and become apparent on eruption. Such teeth are often unsightly or prone to excessive toothwear or loss of clinical crowns, and thus they may require restoration to improve appearance or function or to protect the underlying tooth structure. These defects, their aetiology, and clinical appearance are outlined in Table 2.6, Chapter 2 with examples shown and include the acquired conditions of enamel hypoplasia, molar-incisor hypomineralization and intrinsic staining (fluorosis and tetracycline) as well as the hereditary conditions of hypodontia, amelogenesis imperfecta, and dentinogenesis imperfecta.

1.6 Answers to self-test questions

Q1.5: What habit may have contributed to this pattern of disease?

A: This child was allowed to suck a bottle of sweet drink frequently.

Q1.7: How may this area of the lesion arrested?

A: Improved oral hygiene would have arrested this active part of the lesion.

Q1.8: What ions have contributed to the intact surface zone?

A: Fluoride, calcium, and phosphate ions in particular help to form a more acid-resistant fluoride-substituted hydroxyapatite.

Q1.9: How might this scenario be managed in a high caries risk patient?

A: Instruct the patient regarding their oral hygiene procedures and if this does not improve then carry out debridement/air-abrasion followed by application of a fissure sealant.

Q1.11: What features of this lesion will help the dentist conclude that it is active, how might these be detected, and how might the patient be managed?

A: The lesion has surface roughness (detectable as vibrations in the handle of the ball-ended explorer as it is gently run across the lesion surface) and was covered with plaque (detected visually, disclosing agent). This patient was under preventive therapy including modifications in their oral hygiene, possibly diet, and application of fluoride varnish to arrest the lesion.

Q1.13: What causes the colour change in dentine caries?

A: Not conclusive, but may be due to the Maillard reaction, a biochemical reaction between proteins and carbohydrates in a moist, acidic biological environment.

Q1.15: How many other carious lesions can you detect?

A: Distal/ mesial (d/m) UR6, d/m UR5, m LR7, d/m LR6, d/m LR5, not including the grossly broken down UR4!

Q1.16: What might have been the presenting dental complaints for the above patient?

A: Pain, difficultly chewing, sharp fractured teeth/fillings against the tongue or cheeks, not being able to bite properly, poor appearance, difficulty in brushing the teeth due to sensitivity, and tooth fractures.

Q1.17a: Can you detect any abnormal clinical findings from the above picture?

A: Difficult, but did you notice the mucosal swelling level with the mucogingival junction adjacent to the UL3?

Q1.17c: What other findings are evident from the USO?

A: The near complete obliteration of the pulp chamber and root canal spaces in the UL1.

2

Clinical detection: 'information gathering'

Chapter contents

2.1 Introduction

The dental team (dentist, nurse, hygienist/therapist/oral health educator, laboratory technician, receptionist) led by the principal practitioner, can all be involved in the decision-making processes and dental management of the patient. Sometimes the dentist will refer difficult cases to a specialist dentist for their opinion as to what the diagnosis and care plan should be.

To manage patients successfully, there are five stages that must be followed (see Figure 2.1):

1. Detecting clinical problems and their aetiology (Chapter 2):

   • This involves detective work to help gather clinically relevant and useful information primarily using the skills of verbal history taking, oral examination and relevant special investigations.

2. Diagnosis and risk assessment (Chapter 3):

   • The art of interpretation of signs and symptoms/results from investigations to conclude with identifying the cause of the problem and the potential chance the individual patient has of developing further disease or responding to treatment. Both aspects are critical to planning the overall care of the patient.

3. Prognosis (Chapter 3):

   • The art of forecasting the course of a disease or problem, whether treated or not.

4. Formulating an individualized care plan (treatment plan) (Chapters 3–5):

- An outline of the overall management strategy for the individual patient as well as itemized treatments when required.
- Includes control of disease ('prevention') and/or restoration of teeth when required, using the first principles of minimally invasive dentistry.

5. Recall (Chapter 8):

- Monitoring the treatment provided and the patient's response to assess if knowledge/behavioural adaptations have helped to control and/or prevent disease reoccurrence.

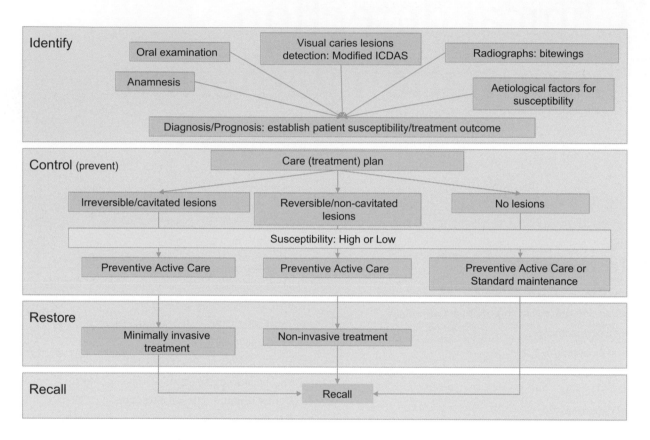

Figure 2.1 Patient care flowchart showing how the patient management stages of *identify* (Chapter 2), *control* (Chapter 4), *restore* (Chapters 5–7), and *recall* (Chapter 8) link to one another. (Adapted from Domejean *et al*. Minimal Intervention Treatment Plan (MITP): practical implementation in general practice. *J Min Intervent Dent* 2009;**2**:103–23.)

2.2 Detection/identification: 'information gathering'

This aspect of patient management involves gathering the relevant information based on which sound clinical judgements can be made as to the best course of treatment for the individual patient. Clinical detection works on two levels:

- Detecting the immediate clinical problem (i.e. the actual manifestation of the disease process, e.g. carious lesions, toothwear (TW) lesions).
- Detecting and understanding the complex interplay of aetiological factors that have *caused* the problem for that particular patient.

It is critical that detailed notes are made for all stages of the patient management pathway, at every visit. This can be done through computer software packages or hand-written notes. Each patient will have his/her own notes with their name, address, contact details, and occupation listed. It is essential to check that the correct notes have been called up for the attending patient and for each visit, the date and time of appointment must be noted initially.

2.3 Taking a verbal history

The art of verbal history taking is the first and one of the most critical ways of obtaining information about any problems the patient may present with and also their aetiology. The answers to a carefully planned series of questions will help to shed light on the nature and severity of the problem presented. A generic structured 'interview' with the clinical relevance of each question is presented in Table 2.1. This, of course, is not the only format of questioning that can be used, and with experience can be adjusted to specific needs and conditions and modified to assess aetiological factors of the presenting disease (see later).

Table 2.1 Structured verbal history ordered to ask relevant questions to help unearth the clues for a diagnosis of the presenting problem and formulating an individualized care plan

Structuring the verbal history	Comments
Patient complains of ... (C/O)	Note down, in the patient's own words, the presenting symptom(s)/problem(s).
History of presenting complaint(s) (HPC)	*Commencement*: when did it start? *Location*: ask patient to describe or ask to point/outline area with one finger. *Type*: description of symptoms. Avoid putting words in the patient's mouth. *Incidence*: how long ago did the episodes start? *Duration*: how long do they persist? Frequency? Are they getting better, staying the same or deteriorating? *Initiating/relieving factors*: does anything make the symptoms worse or better? Answers to the above will often provide the clues to help make the correct diagnosis.
Past dental history (PDH)	What previous dental treatment have they experienced (orthodontics/extractions/perio, etc). How regularly do they visit the dentist? What previous preventive advice have they received/do they follow? These answers will enable the dentist to create a picture of the attitude/motivation of the patient towards dentistry and their own oral health, without asking them directly about these issues.
Medical history (MH)	Most dentists use a printed checklist, which should include information regarding: • Cardiac problems/disease/rheumatic fever/blood pressure • Respiratory disease/asthma/shortness of breath • Diabetes/epilepsy/jaundice /hepatitis history • Current/recent past medications • Allergies • Bleeding/haemorrhage/clotting defects • Other illnesses/operations/hospital admissions • Pregnancy • HIV/AIDS risk. Information relevant regarding drug interactions with local anaesthetic, allergies to latex/resins/dental materials. Bleeding problems/anticoagulant therapies relevant for periodontal surgery, root planing, extractions. Check medication in the *Dental Formulary* or equivalent. Medications causing dry mouth, gingival overgrowth, or vomiting should be noted.
Social history (SH)	Occupation/family members/availability for appointments. Relevant when considering appointment logistics for the care plan for the individual.
Habits	Oral hygiene (OH – procedures, frequency), diet (amount/frequency of sugar intake, balanced diet, erosive potential for toothwear), smoking, alcohol intake, parafunctional habits (bruxism (teeth grinding), clenching). Relevant when planning care, preventive advice. What the patient says might be checked/verified during the oral examination to follow. Helps to ascertain the possible aetiology of the problem.

2

2.4 Physical examination

Once the verbal history has been taken, a physical examination follows, divided into a general and oral examination.

General examination

This will commence as the dentist interviews the patient. The demeanour of the individual, facial/optical asymmetries, facial nerve palsies, pallor, tremors, or mental/physical disabilities can be noted and followed up if relevant to the dental treatment required.

Oral examination (Table 2.2)

A common error made by inexperienced dental undergraduates is to dive into an oral examination and direct all attention immediately to the teeth. It is better to have a system that encompasses all aspects of oral health including the soft tissues and periodontal tissues, as well as teeth and prostheses. When examining the oral mucosae, learn a system which ensures that all aspects of the oral cavity are included, i.e. front to back (lips to tonsils), back to front or clockwise/anticlockwise around the oral cavity . Once learnt, this is never forgotten, even during the stress of clinical examinations! Ensure adequate time has been set aside for the examination along with suitable dental instrumentation (Chapter 5).

Table 2.2 Steps in a comprehensive oral examination. Note that a full examination should not be rushed and careful recording of findings is essential

Examination site		Comments
Extraoral		Facial swellings/asymmetries, lips – form and seal, facial and neck lymph nodes, TMJ – crepitus, clicking (uni-bilateral), mandibular movement (opening gape, deviations, lateral/protrusive excursions). Operator stands behind the patient for the TMJ/LN exam – remember to warn the patient prior to starting!
Intra-oral	**Mucosae**	All internal buccal, labial, alveolar mucosae including vermilion border of lips, tongue (dorsum, lateral borders and ventral surfaces), retromolar areas, hard and soft palate, floor of mouth. Palpation of the pterygoid muscles. Checking for white or erythematous patches/plaques indicative of trauma, lichenoid reactions, neoplastic change – referral to an oral medicine specialist might be appropriate. Tenderness in the pterygoids muscles – ? sign of TMD. Dry mucosae and frothy saliva indicative of dry mouth.
	Periodontium	Marginal gingivae (colour, contour, consistency), gingivitis (BPE score), recession, loss of attachment, probing depths, mobility, presence of supra-/subgingival calculus, plaque indices. Relevant to assess periodontal status, which will affect the overall restorative status of the mouth and of the individual tooth.
	Teeth	Missing teeth, mobility, restoration status, caries, toothwear (site, enamel ± dentine), malpositioning (tilting, rotation, overeruption/submerged).
	Prostheses	Crowns, removable dentures, fixed bridges, implant-retained crown and bridge work, orthodontic appliances (fixed and removable). Relevant regarding oral hygiene procedures, plaque-retentive margins, aesthetics, status of abutment teeth.
	Occlusion	Angle's classification (Class I, II, III), incisor relationship (Class I, II division 1/2 and Class III). Intercuspal position (ICP), retruded contact position (RCP), protrusive, retrusive, lateral excursive movements – working and non-working side contacts. Skeletal discrepancies. Relevant to the restoration of individual/groups of teeth to conform to existing occlusal harmony or to assess changes in a reorganized approach in more complex treatment plans (Chapter 5).

TMJ, temporomandibular joint; LN, lymph node; TMD, temporomandibular dysfunction; BPE, basic periodontal examination.

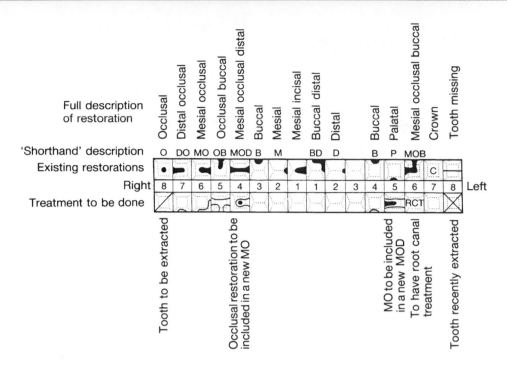

Figure 2.2 Conventions for recording restorations, lesions/teeth requiring restoration, teeth to be extracted and other conditions on a dental chart.

Q2.2: Can you spot an error in the above charting?

2.4.1 Dental charting

When examining the dentition, there are certain features that the dentist must relay to his/her nurse to record accurately in a dental chart (see Figure 2.2). This chart is interpreted as though the dentist is looking at a patient face to face and the notation is communicated from the patient's perspective.

1. Which tooth, side, position – e.g. 'upper left 6' or 'upper left first permanent molar', rotated/tilted/space-closed.

2. Presence of existing restoration(s) – location (mesio-occlusal, buccal, cervical, etc.) and type of material (amalgam, tooth-coloured, gold, ceramic, etc).

3. Status of existing restorations – sound, or deficient margins/fractured/missing.

4. Presence of carious lesion(s) – location, mICDAS classification (see later), lesion activity.

5. Presence of toothwear – location (buccal, occlusal, incisal) and extent (in enamel or dentine, exposing pulp)

6. Presence of other abnormalities, e.g. fluorosis, hypoplastic enamel, cracks.

With practice, this can be done with a series of abbreviated responses, and good teamwork with the nurse can expedite this process. Of course, if above points 2–6 do not apply after careful examination, then a summary of 'sound' will usually suffice and a dot is placed on the relevant tooth in the chart. It is important to check all five surfaces of each tooth either with direct vision or using the dental mirror and good lighting of a clean tooth. It might be necessary in some patients, before the visual examination (but after checking any relevant medical history), to clean the dentition with a periodontal hand/ultrasonic scaler in order to remove supragingival plaque and calculus deposits that might be obscuring clear view of the tooth surfaces.

2.4.2 Tooth notation

In the UK, the most commonly used notations are the Palmer system and a two-letter coding system. Both are shown in Figure 2.3, dividing the mouth into four quadrants with the teeth in each numbered 1–8 from central incisors to third molars:

A drawback of the Palmer notation is that this can be difficult to input into electronic notes (although current software packages are accommodating this system).

UR	8	7	6	5	4	3	2	1		1	2	3	4	5	6	7	8	UL
LR	8	7	6	5	4	3	2	1		1	2	3	4	5	6	7	8	LL

Figure 2.3 The Palmer and two-letter coding system (UR, upper right; UL, upper left; LR, lower right; LL, lower left) communicated as thought the dentist is looking directly at the patient. In both systems the deciduous dentition is labelled a–e from the midline.

UR	18 17 16 15 14 13 12 11	21 22 23 24 25 26 27 28	UL
LR	48 47 46 45 44 43 42 41	31 32 33 34 35 36 37 38	LL

Figure 2.4 The FDI tooth notation system with the teeth in each quadrant prefixed by a number 1–4.

UR	1 2 3 4 5 6 7 8	9 10 11 12 13 14 15 16	UL
LR	32 31 30 29 28 27 26 25	24 23 22 21 20 19 18 17	LL

Figure 2.5 The Universal tooth notation system, with each individual tooth being allocated a number from 1 to 32 in the permanent dentition.

2.5 Caries detection

Visual detection of carious lesions in enamel and dentine relies on the following operator-controlled factors:

- Using 'sharp' eyes and the possible use of magnification in the form of dental loupes (Chapter 5).
- Using good illumination from the overhead dental chair light or a more focused light from a fibreoptic headlight coupled with the use of loupes.
- Having clean tooth surfaces to examine, both wet and dry (using a 3-1 air/water syringe). If surface debris (plaque/calculus) is present

Two numerical notation systems exist: the FDI (Federation Dentaire Internationale – favoured in mainland Europe; see Figure 2.4) and the Universal system (favoured in the USA; see Figure 2.5). Users tend to credit these systems for crossing language boundaries but confusion can occur easily with these solely numerical notations, e.g. FDI 16 (see Figure 2.4) represents UR6 (upper right first permanent molar, 6⌋), whereas Universal 16 (see Figure 2.5) represents UL8 (upper left third permanent molar, ⌊8).

this may have to be removed prior to any dental examination taking place (see Figure 2.6).

- Using blunt dental explorers – the use of sharp dental probes is contraindicated for carious lesion detection as they can potentially cause cavitation in a previously non-cavitated lesion (see Figure 2.7).
- Sufficient time allocated for the examination of all tooth surfaces as well as the soft tissues and periodontium.

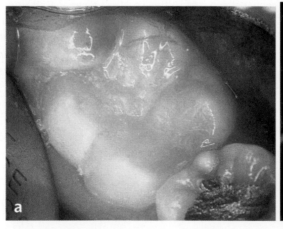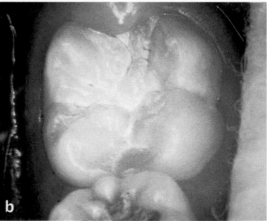

Figure 2.6 (**a**) Apparently caries-free occlusal surface of an erupting molar. (**b**) Thorough debridement, washing, and drying reveals white spot lesions in the occlusal fissures. An example of mICDAS 1 – see later. (Courtesy of *Dental Update*.)

Q2.6: What is the name given to the overlying segment of gingivae on the distal aspect of the occlusal surface in both examples above?

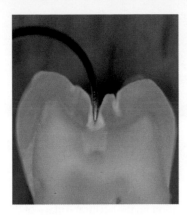

Figure 2.7 A cross-section of a tooth through a demineralized enamel fissure showing the damage inflicted to the intact enamel bridge at the tip of the sharp dental explorer – use of sharp probes is contraindicated for caries detection (courtesy of Professor E Reich).

Q2.7: What hand instrument should be used instead?

2.5.1 Indices

The histopathology and clinical signs of the carious lesion have been described in Chapter 1. The clinical manifestation of the carious disease process is the progressive lesion it creates within the dental hard tissues. A dentist must be able to link the visual clinical appearance of the lesion with the underlying histological damage that has occurred in the tooth, at a particular moment in time. In this way, the dentist can then decide how to manage the lesion and the disease process in that individual patient. In an attempt to do this, several visual indices have been described over the years. In 2004, the ICDAS (International Caries Detection and Assessment System) Foundation was convened to produce an evidence-based clinical caries assessment system to be used primarily for epidemiological and research studies, as well as for use in general dental practice. A simpler, modified version is presented in Table 2.3 with clinical examples (see Figures 2.8–2.10), which permits the dentist to examine clinically the tooth surface and appreciate the underlying damage that has been caused. Then, depending on the individual's caries risk assessment, the most relevant treatment option can be chosen. This index requires that points listed and discussed

2

Table 2.3 A modified ICDAS (mICDAS) carious lesion scoring system (0–4), linking the clinical appearance (black text) with the equivalent underlying lesion histology (red text). Images show teeth sectioned longitudinally through occlusal lesions, representative clinical examples of each mICDAS score. This clinical scoring system is useful for inclusion in the patient's notes, monitoring, and medicolegal purposes

0		No or slight change in enamel translucency after prolonged air drying (>5 s). No enamel demineralization or a narrow surface zone of opacity.
1		Opacity or discoloration from the enamel (white spot lesion) hardly visible on a wet surface, but distinctly visible after air drying. No cavitation on occlusal/smooth surfaces. Enamel demineralization limited to outer 50%.
2		Enamel opacity (white spot lesion) or greyish discoloration distinctly visible without the need for air drying. No clinical cavitation detectable. Demineralization involving inner 50% of enamel through to the outer third of dentine.
3		Localized enamel breakdown in opaque or discolored enamel, ± greyish discoloration/shadowing from underlying dentine. Demineralization involving the middle to inner third of dentine.
4		Gross cavitation in opaque or discolored enamel exposing the underlying stained dentine. Demineralization involving the inner third of dentine towards pulp.

2

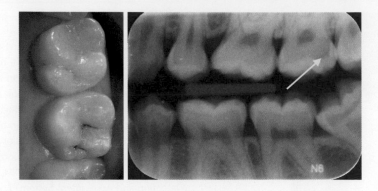

Figure 2.8 The brown, non-cavitated fissures with underlying grey discoloration on the occlusal surface of the UL7 are caused by demineralized, discoloured dentine shining through intact, wet enamel (a closed lesion, visible in dentine on the bitewing radiograph (right, yellow arrow) – mICDAS 2).

Q2.8: What treatment may be required for this tooth?

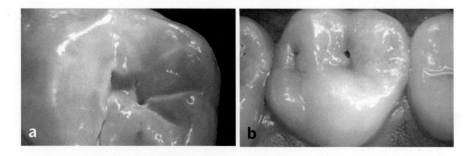

Figure 2.9 (**a**, **b**) A small cavity is just detectable within the whitish opacity/brown discoloration on the occlusal surfaces of these molars, appearing as a widened fissure and a cavitated pit respectively. They can easily be missed clinically unless the surfaces are clean and vision aided by the use of magnification. Histologically, both lesions were well into dentine, visible on radiographs – mICDAS 3.

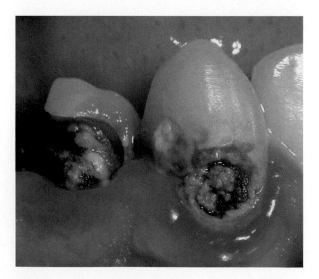

Figure 2.10 Grossly cavitated buccal carious lesions on LR3 and 4 with quantities of stagnant dense plaque deposited on the exposed dentine – mICDAS 4.

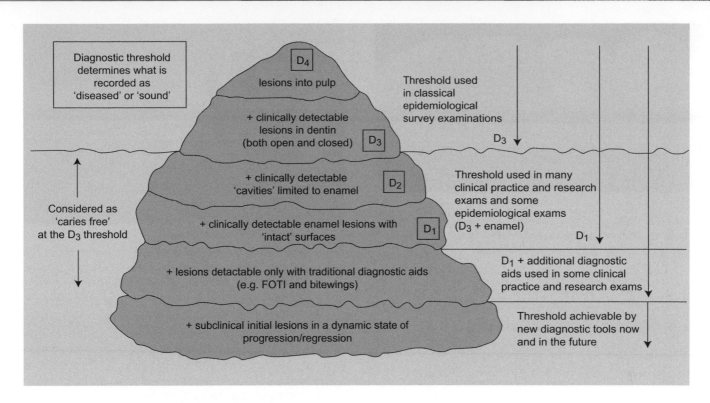

Figure 2.11 The caries iceberg classifying clinically detectable lesions with regard to their level of tissue invasion and degree of cavitation. FOTI, fibreoptic transillumination. (From Pitts NB (1997). Diagnostic tools and measurements – impact on appropriate care. *Community Dent Oral Epidemiol* **25**:24–35.)

above are carried out judiciously and permits an objective numerical record to be made in the dental chart to permit longitudinal assessment of the particular lesion over time.

Alternative indices exist classifying carious lesions. The 'caries iceberg', developed in collaboration with cariologists and epidemiologists, is an index used by many experts to study the incidence and prevalence of the disease in different populations. This permits the development of strategies to manage caries at a population level as well as at a patient level. The iceberg can be seen in Figure 2.11: clinically detectable

lesions are divided into four groups, D1–D4, depending on the depth of tissue invasion and the degree of cavitation. Note that careful selection of caries detection thresholds is required or else this index may lead to threshold bias when interpreting data for caries prevalence in a population. For example, if D3 detection threshold (dentine lesions, cavitated or not (open or closed)) is selected to establish the presence/absence of caries, patients with early stage lesions within enamel, cavitated or not, will not be included in the final data, thus incorrectly reducing the caries prevalence for that particular population.

2.5.2 Susceptible surfaces

Carious lesions occur on tooth surfaces that have accumulated plaque and this has been allowed to stagnate for a prolonged period of time:

- The depths of pits and fissures on posterior occlusal surfaces (which cannot be cleaned effectively with a tooth brush). These areas on newly erupting, partially erupted or submerged molars are particularly susceptible to carious attack.
- Proximal surfaces (mesial and distal) *cervical* to contact points of adjacent teeth (where patients may not floss regularly/at all). The surfaces of particularly imbricated (crowded) teeth can be more susceptible due to the lack of access to oral hygiene aids.

- Smooth surfaces adjacent to the gingival margin (again where patients often miss with their tooth brush).
- The ledged/overhanging margins of restorations (a plaque trap often inaccessible to a tooth brush/floss).

Of course, these are not the only sites on which carious lesions occur. The site and distribution of lesions in a patient's mouth might give an indication to underlying aetiological factors. For example, patients with xerostomia (dry mouth) due to salivary gland disease or damage (for example, from radiotherapy when treating head and neck cancers) can develop lesions on the incisal surfaces of anterior teeth and lesions that circumvent the neck of the crown at the gingival margin. Patients with eating disorders may have lesions on the lingual-cervical aspect of the mandibular teeth (see Figure 2.12).

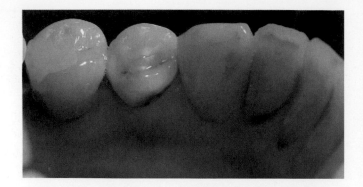

Figure 2.12 A patient with an eating disorder, anorexia nervosa, with carious cavitated lesions on the lingual aspects of LL124 (mICDAS 2,3).

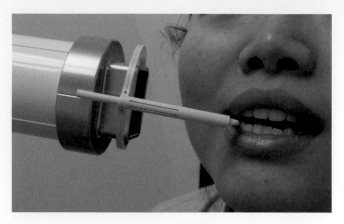

Figure 2.13 Right bitewing radiograph being taken with film holder and beam-aiming device (yellow arm) enabling optimal alignment of the radiographic beam at right angles to the teeth and intraoral film.

2.5.3 Special investigations

To aid the process of clinical information gathering, other tests may be requested, the results of which must help verify or make the final diagnosis of the problem and possibly its aetiology. Investigations have a cost implication to the patient or the health service provider and depending on the test, may be invasive or even potentially harmful in nature. It is imperative that information gathered using multiple special investigations must not be interpreted individually, but in conjunction with all the other methods described in this chapter to help formulate the diagnosis for the patient. All investigations are prone to false-positive and false-negative outcomes. Analysing the relative proportions of these outcomes, statistical measures of *sensitivity* (the measure of how effective an investigation is at detecting true disease) and *specificity* (the measure of how effective an investigation is at detecting true health) can be developed, which are useful in assessing the investigation's value in providing a suitable diagnostic yield. For caries detection, these include radiographs and pulp vitality (sensibility) and percussion tests.

Radiographs

Horizontal bitewing radiographs should be used to aid lesion detection on proximal surfaces of posterior teeth especially when adjacent teeth are present and direct vision is not possible. A film holder and beam-aiming device should be used routinely in order to obtain the optimal angulation of the beam perpendicular to the contact points and to allow reproducibility of films when monitoring lesions over a period of time (see Figure 2.13).

Incipient occlusal lesions are difficult to detect and only later stage occlusal lesions are clearly visible on radiographs. Periapical radiographs may be used to assess the depth of proximal lesions in anterior teeth. Dental panoramic tomograms should not be routinely used for caries detection due to their limited resolution and increased radiation dose when compared with small intraoral films. The radiographic appearance of caries (a radiolucency in enamel or dentine) is often described as being up to six months behind the actual histological spread of the lesion in the tooth. Therefore, a lesion radiographically restricted to enamel will probably have spread histologically across the enamel–dentine junction (EDJ) into the outer third of dentine.

Table 2.4 shows how the mICDAS scores for the visual and histological lesion appearance correlate with the radiographic appearance/depth of enamel and dentine lesions. Examples of lesions detected from bitewing radiographs of a high caries risk patient are shown in Figure 2.14. Once experience has been gained in interpreting radiographs, other clues can often be found to help with the diagnosis and potential activity status of the lesion(s). These might include the outline of the pulp horns – often tertiary dentine has been laid down in response to the disease process and this can be seen by the relative shrinkage of the pulp horn subjacent to the spreading lesion. Also, the 'moth eaten' appearance of the advancing edge of the radiolucency is a clue that, at the time when the film was taken, the lesion was in a state of relative activity causing demineralization. If the dentine–pulp complex has had a chance to lay down extra mineral to 'wall off' the lesion (a more defined radio-opaque boundary), this implies a relative tip in the metabolic balance towards healing.

It is vital that a report of all radiographic findings is duly noted in the patient's notes for long-term scrutiny, monitoring, and medicolegal reasons.

Table 2.4 The association between the radiographic lesion depth (E1–D3) and equivalent mICDAS scores

Enamel Lesion		mICDAS
EI	Outer half of enamel	0, 1
E2	Inner half of enamel	1
Dentine Lesion		**mICDAS**
D1	Outer third of dentine	2
D2	Middle third of dentine	3
D3	Inner third of dentine	4

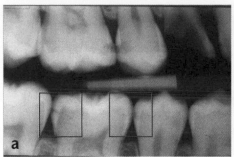
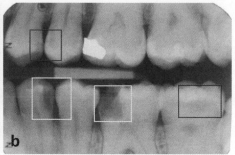

Figure 2.14 (**a**) Right and (**b**) left bitewing radiographs from two different patients both with high caries experience, showing carious lesions within enamel and outer third dentine (E2–D1, blue square), approaching middle third of dentine (D2, red square) and very close to the pulp (D3, yellow square) Note, other lesions can be detected on these films.

Q2.14: Can you find more lesions and radiographically classify them? Can you comment on the radiographic changes of the pulp chambers in those teeth?

Pulp vitality (sensibility) tests

Technically, the term vitality implies the status of the pulpal blood flow. This can be measured using laser Doppler flowmetry, which has mainly been applied for research purposes. Clinical signs of a non-vital, necrotic pulp may include:

- Discoloration and darkening of the tooth due to the breakdown products of haemoglobin in the pulp chamber. Greying and reduced translucency might also be noticed. These changes may be difficult to detect if the tooth is heavily restored or has an extracoronal restoration covering it.

- Over time, a necrotic pulp may give rise to a sinus tracking from the periapical tissues to the mucosal surface usually adjacent to the apex of the tooth in question. A fine gutta percha point inserted into the endodontic sinus and then radiographed will show the direction of the sinus track and ultimately the periapical origin of the infection (see Figure 2.15).

The status of pulp innervation (sensibility) can be assessed to ascertain the effect of the carious process on the tooth:

- *Temperature*: heat from warm gutta percha sticks (rare) or cold from cotton wool pledgets soaked in ethyl chloride or ice sticks may be used to ascertain the status of pulpal innervation. Tooth surfaces to be assessed must be dry and clear of surface debris (plaque/calculus; see Figure 2.16). Check equivalent teeth on the contralateral side to the tooth in question and then the adjacent teeth (acting as an internal control), ensuring the cotton wool/ice stick/gutta percha is placed on a clean, dry, sound tooth surface. Ask the patient to raise a hand when they feel a sensation in the tooth being tested. Vital teeth tend to respond quickly, whereas false-positive readings respond more slowly (conduction through dentine/metallic restoration into the periodontal membrane).

- *Electrical*: a mono-polar electric pulp tester passes a small current (direct or alternating) through the patient and the tooth it is in contact with. The patient's hand must be in contact with the metal

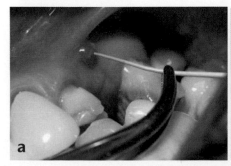
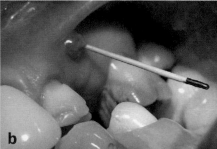
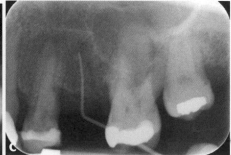

Figure 2.15 (**a**) A soft, non-tender swelling on the dentoalveolar mucosa distally adjacent to the periapical region of the broken-down UL4, a chronic sinus, into which a sterile gutta percha point has been carefully inserted (**b**) and radiograph showing the exact location of the 'abscess' (**c**). The UL6 is vital with no symptoms.

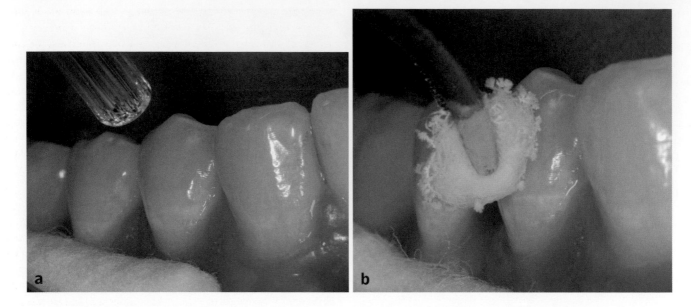

Figure 2.16 (**a**) Pulp sensibility testing of cleaned and air-dried LR4 using cold ethyl chloride-soaked cotton wool pledget (**b**). Avoid restorations and the gingival margin as false-positive readings may ensue.

handle of the handpiece to complete the circuit with some units. The probe is placed on a clean, sound tooth surface (contralateral and adjacent equivalents tested first as an internal patient control) using an electrolytic coupling agent on the tooth surface to ensure completion of the circuit (usually a small amount of prophylaxis paste; see Figure 2.17). The current is gradually increased by the dentist until the patient feels a tingling sensation in the tooth. At this point they are instructed to let go of the handpiece and the circuit is broken. The numerical value can be recorded and is useful for monitoring purposes for a particular tooth but is not equivocal as the readings can vary from the same patient. False-positive responses may be elicited through stimulation of nerve fibres in the periodontium and in posterior multirooted teeth, a mixture of vital and non-vital pulp tissue may confound the interpretation of the reading.

- *Cutting a test cavity without local anaesthesia*: a rarely used, last resort method that checks the innervation of the dentine–pulp complex by drilling vital dentine. If the patient feels pain then at least partial innervation of the pulp remains.

It is important to note in the above cases, a positive response from the pulp does not necessarily mean all is well. There is no clinical way of knowing if there is partial necrosis or denervation in a dental pulp and multirooted teeth can present with partially diseased pulpal tissue.

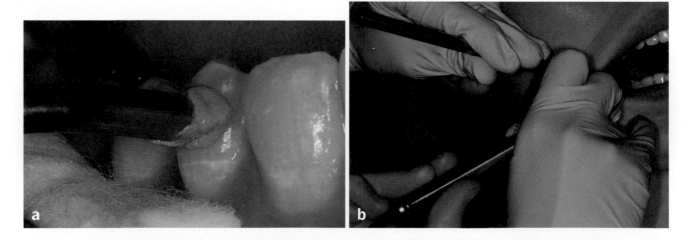

Figure 2.17 (**a**) Probe of the electric pulp tester placed on clean dry tooth surface, coupled with prophypaste. (**b**) Note the patient's fingers (un-gloved) touching the probe handle so completing the electrical circuit. They should let go to break the circuit when a sensation is felt in the tooth.

Percussion tests

Percussion tests (gently tapping the crown axially and then obliquely with a probe or mirror handle) assess the physical condition of the periapical tissues and periodontal membrane, not the pulp directly. If periapical periodontitis is present, the piston-like effect of the tooth being pushed into the inflamed periapical tissues will elicit acute tenderness. The inflammation in the periodontal tissues might be caused by the toxins from a non-vital pulp.

2.5.4 Lesion activity – risk assessment

Once a carious lesion is detected, it would also be useful to ascertain whether it is currently active (the disease process is ongoing) or inactive in order for the correct care plan to be implemented. This is difficult to measure objectively intraorally, but certain intraoral clues can be gleaned from the:

- *Colour and surface texture of a cavitated lesion*: an arrested lesion is often darker in colour and the exposed dentine has a flint-like, hard, shiny outer surface when probed.
- *Presence of gingival bleeding on the same tooth*: the presence of a gingival inflammatory reaction implies poor oral hygiene in that area, which will increase the risk of plaque accumulation.
- *Presence of plaque*: if a biofilm is overlying the lesion, it can reasonably be assumed to be in a state of activity as it is the presence of the plaque biofilm that is critical to the development of the carious lesion (see Figure 2.18a). If plaque can be found on non-retentive sites, again this implies poor oral hygiene measures and therefore an increased risk of caries incidence.
- *Accessibility to OH procedures*: if lesions are present in uncleansable sites (see earlier) then again it is likely that the lesions will be active as a biofilm will remain on their surfaces.
- *Use of plaque indicators* (see Figure 2.18b,c): dental manufacturers have produced two- or even three-tone plaque disclosing solutions,

which can give the dentist and patient an indication not only on which surfaces the plaque biofilm is stagnating, but also for how long, as well as the plaque density. The bacterial population (and the cariogenicity) of the biofilm develops in a structured manner in correlation with its age – the older the plaque, the more anaerobic and acidic the conditions on the enamel surface are likely to be. These proprietary kits neither assess the direct activity of lesions nor patient susceptibility to caries from the relative quantities, age and acidogenicity of plaque, but can usefully add to all the other information gathered from the history and examination, so helping to formulate an overall picture of the individual's susceptibility to caries. They also can be helpful as strong motivators for patients to improve their own oral health with better oral hygiene procedures.

- *Use of saliva tests*: The absence of saliva or the presence of a reduced quality of saliva is an important aetiological factor in the increased susceptibility of patients to the disease. Volumetric and flow rate analyses can be carried out using chairside kits and crude levels of *mutans streptococci* (an indicator of the carious process) can also be calculated. If the results of volumetric/flow rate analyses are low and there are high levels of *Streptococcus mutans* in a sample of the patient's saliva, then, *in conjunction with the results of other clinical investigations*, the dentist may collate evidence that points to the patient having a higher caries risk, and the lesions present having an increased chance of being active.

2.5.5 Diet analysis

The primary aetiological factors for dental caries, as described in Chapter 1, are a susceptible tooth surface, presence of bacteria, fermentable carbohydrates, and enough time for the combination to start demineralizing the tooth surface within the plaque biofilm. The surfaces of the teeth can be examined for carious lesions, as can the bacterial levels in plaque and saliva (see above). The other main aetiological factor that can be assessed during this detection phase of patient management, is

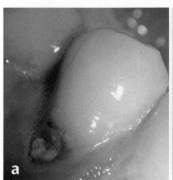
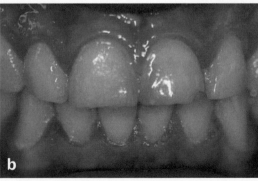
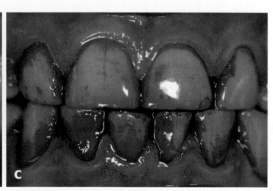

Figure 2.18 (**a**) Plaque biofilm sitting on the surface of a buccal cervical carious lesion indicating its potential activity. (**b**) Anterior view of dentition with a 36-hour accumulation of plaque. (**c**) A two-tone plaque indicator applied (dark blue and pink), highlighting the differing densities of plaque accumulated on the labial and gingival margins of the same teeth in (**b**).

Q2.18a: How could you manage this case?

dietary intake of refined carbohydrate and sugar levels in patients exhibiting signs of high caries risk (multiple lesions (>2) developed within the previous two years). This is done by asking the patient to fill out a diet analysis sheet (see Figure 2.19) usually over a period of at least three days, encompassing Saturday and/or Sunday. They should be advised to write down everything that passes between their lips in that time (including water, numbers of spoons of sugar in tea/coffee, etc.) and to note when they brush their teeth.

No indication of the relevance of the diet analysis should be given at the first appointment so as not to bias the patient or allow them to cheat by writing down a diet intake they feel is an improvement on what they are actually doing! The results should then be analysed by the dentist and an appointment made to discuss them. Issues to look out for are frequency of meals, hidden sugar content (e.g. many sauces are high in sugar), medications, drinks (additional sugar/high sugar content/erosive potential due to high titratable acidity). It is imperative that the dentist works with the patient to *modify* their existing dietary habits. Chastising the patient and ordering them to change may have the opposite effect! Work with positive reinforcement, offering suggestions or allowing the patient to make sensible suggestions to lower their sugar intake, frequency, and duration. Remember, positive encouragement of small changes over time are most likely to get positive results.

2.5.6 Caries detection technologies

As an adjunct to the principles and methods describe above, there are other technologies available to help the dentist detect carious lesions. Examples of some of these are shown in Table 2.5. Many detection technologies work on four basic physical principles affecting mineralized dental tissues: optical light scattering, mineral density changes, fluorescent characteristics and tissue porosity. It is important to understand how a particular technology works to be able to interpret accurately the information it is giving. An example of such an ambiguity is the DiagnoDent laser-fluorescence caries detection system. Note that in Table 2.5, this system has been placed into two categories, optical light scattering and fluorescent characteristics, as research has shown the unit is affected by both properties to a varying degree. Therefore the interpretation of results, that is whether to cut a cavity or not, must be used with caution in the clinical environment, again in conjunction with all the other information gathered for the particular patient.

	Thursday			Friday			Saturday			Sunday		
	Time	Item	🙂	Time	Item	🙂	Time	Item	🙂	Time	Item	🙂
Before breakfast	7.30	Tea*		7.0	Tea*		7.30	Tea*		7.05	Tea*	
Breakfast	8.00	2 Wheat slices 2 Crisp bread 1 Apple Coffee*		8.00	2 Wheat slices 2 Crisp bread 1 Apple Coffee*		8.30	2 Wheat slices 2 Crisp bread 1 Apple Coffee*		8.05	2 Wheat slices 2 Crispbread 1 Apple Coffee*	
Morning	9.00	Polo		10.00 / 11.30	Murray mint / Tea* Biscuit		11.15	Tea*		10.00 / 12.30	Lemon Barley / Tea*	
Mid-day Meal	12.30	Meat roll Tea*		2.00	Steamed fish Parsley sauce Boiled potatoes		1.45	Sausage, onion, Boiled potatoes Ice Cream, tinned fruit		1.40	Roast lamb, potatoes, cabbage, carrots	
Afternoon	2.00 / 5.30	2 Cream crackers 1 Dairy Lea Tea* / 2 Shortbread biscuits Tea*		2.45 / 6.00	Tea* / Tea*		2.30 / 5.45	Tea* / Tea*		2.00 / 4.00	Tea* / Tea*	
Evening Meal	8.00	Chop, leeks, boiled potatoes Choc-ice Tea*		8.30	Bacon sandwich Tea*		7.30	Fried kipper bread and butter		8.15	Ham salad, bread and butter Tea*	
Evening and night	1.00	Horlicks* Biscuits		10.00 / 1.30	Peanuts / Horlicks* Biscuit		9.15 / 1.45	Chocolate / Horlicks* Biscuits		1.15	Horlicks* Biscuits	

Figure 2.19 Diet analysis sheet filled in by a middle-aged man with a high incidence of caries.

Q2.19: What stands out as the main problem regarding this patient's sugar intake?

Table 2.5 Examples of modern technologies available to help detect and characterize carious lesions. The four columns indicate the basic physical principle on which each technology relies. The second row gives the technologies useful in the research laboratory

	OPTICAL/ LIGHT SCATTERING	MINERAL DENSITY	FLUORESCENCE	TISSUE POROSITY
In Vivo	Modified ICDAS classification Fibreoptic transillumination UV illumination Quantitative laser fluorescence (QLF) DiagnoDent	Radiography (digital) Radio VisioGraphy Computer tomography (CT) scans (Cone Beam)	Quantitative laser fluorescence Dye-enhanced laser fluorescence UV illumination DiagnoDent	Electrical Conductance Measurement (ECM) AC Impedance Dye-enhanced laser fluorescence Dye penetration (iodide) Ultrasound
In Vitro	Polarized, transmitted light microscopy (PTLM) Spectroscopy (IR, microRaman) Reflected light confocal microscopy	SEM Quantitative back-scattered SEM Microradiography Microfocal CT X-ray microtomography X-ray microanalysis	Confocal laser-scanning fluorescence microscopy	Polarized transmission Light microscopy Acoustic microscopy

2.6 Toothwear (TW) – clinical detection

2.6.1 Targeted verbal history

In patients with toothwear lesions, it is vital that not only are these detected and a putative cause attributed (i.e. erosive, attritive or abrasive lesions from their clinical presentation – see later), but also that the aetiology of the erosion/attrition/abrasion is appreciated by both the patient and the dentist. In this way, the overall clinical problem can be successfully managed. Coupled to the general information obtained from the initial history as discussed previously, more specific questions may be targeted to assess the aetiology of the specific type of toothwear, often after the initial clinical examination:

● Relating to erosion:

  – Past/present diet (using a diet analysis sheet (see Figure 2.19); questions regarding specific acidic food/drinks using an *aide mémoire* (see Figure 2.20)

  – Digestive disorders causing regurgitation erosion/pregnancy sickness

  – Past/present slimming habits, eating disorders, periods of weight loss

  – Past/present alcohol intake

  – Past/present medications (e.g. vitamin C, iron preparations)

  – Past/present occupation – ? industrial erosion, rare nowadays.

● Relating to attrition:

  – Clenching/grinding habits – day or night time

  – Levels of stress/anxiety in personal/professional life

  – Evidence of masseteric hypertrophy.

● Relating to abrasion:

  – Past/present oral hygiene techniques (tooth brushing, flossing, abrasive pastes).

  – Habits causing dental abrasion – pipe smoking, pen chewing, fingernail biting, etc. (see Figure 2.24).

Name .... Number .... Sex M F
Address .... Tel no ....
.... Occupation ....
.... Work place ....
Interests, hobbies, sport activities ....
Medication ....
Illness present .... Illness past ....
Has the illness been treated .... By a doctor .... In hospital ....

GASTRIC SYMPTOMS	PAST SYMPTOMS			NO	PRESENT SYMPTOMS		
	Frequency per week	Frequency per day	Duration		Frequency per week	Frequency per day	Duration
Belching							
Heartburn							
Acid taste in the mouth							
Vomiting							
Regurgitation ? chew cud							
Stomach ache							
Gastric pain on awakening							
How does the patient treat gastric pain?							

DIET	PAST CONSUMPTION			NO	PRESENT CONSUMPTION		
	Frequency per week	Frequency per day	Duration		Frequency per week	Frequency per day	Duration
Citrus fruits							
Citrus fruit juice							
Other juices							
Special juices							
Sport drinks							
Fruit berries							
Soft drinks, acidic beverages							
Yoghurt							
Vitamin-C drinks, chewable tablets							
Acid sweets							
Special diet							
Vinegar							
Herb tea							
Pickles							
Other acidic food, etc.							
Alcohol							

Figure 2.20 An example of an *aide mémoire* for use when taking a targeted history for dental erosion.

2.6.2 Clinical presentations of toothwear

The causes of pathological toothwear (erosion, attrition, abrasion, and abfraction) have been discussed in Chapter 1. The clinical examination outlined above will permit visual detection of some characteristic features (site/shape of facets/presence of facets on opposing teeth) of the different presentations of toothwear. However, these are often combined as the cause and, therefore, the clinical manifestations, of toothwear lesions are multifactorial (see Figure 2.21).

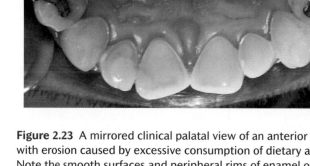

Figure 2.23 A mirrored clinical palatal view of an anterior dentition with erosion caused by excessive consumption of dietary acids. Note the smooth surfaces and peripheral rims of enamel on UL3 to UR3 as well as the amalgam restorations in the premolars standing proud of the tooth surfaces. There was no evidence of gastro-oesophageal reflux from the history.

- *Erosion*: depending on the cause, affects the labial (dietary acids) and palatal smooth surfaces/mandibular buccal/occlusal surfaces (gastric regurgitation acids). Enamel loses surface characterization and becomes smooth (see Figures 2.22, 2.23) and eventually grossly dissolves to expose dentine. Can cause smooth-cupped lesions on posterior occlusal surfaces.
- *Attrition*: often produces sharp, well-defined, interdigitating toothwear lesions on the incisal edges of anterior teeth that meet in occlusion (see Figure 2.22). Can also affect the occlusal surfaces of the molars but to a lesser extent.
- *Abrasion*: lesions caused by repetitive foreign body contact, e.g. toothbrushing (classical v-shaped notching on the buccal cervical aspect of mainly anterior teeth). Can you guess the cause of the abrasion lesions in Figure 2.24?

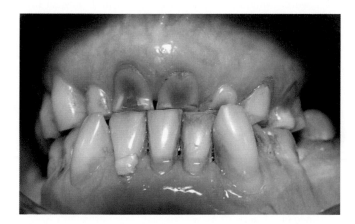

Figure 2.21 A clinical case of toothwear showing the multifactorial aetiology including incisal attrition, labial erosion, and buccal cervical abrasion in a middle-aged patient.

Q2.21: What would be the obvious cause of the buccal cervical abrasion?

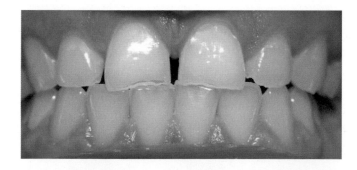

Figure 2.22 A clinical anterior view of a patient with labial-cervical erosion. Note the reflective, smooth, featureless labial enamel surfaces of UR2 to UL2. There are early signs of incisal attrition and resulting blue-grey translucency.

Q2.22: What might be the presenting complaint of this patient?

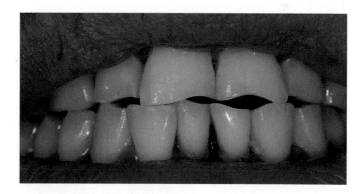

Figure 2.24 An intriguing case of anterior, incisal, undulating abrasion lesions.

Q2.24: What is the cause?

2.6.3 Summary of clinical manifestations of toothwear

- The clinical features of faceting/loss of mineralized tissues highlighted in the previous section, cuspal wear.
- Dental sensitivity/pain caused by rapidly progressing toothwear as dentine tubules are freshly exposed and pain is elicited on hot and cold stimulation (physiological principles of Brannström's hydrodynamic theory). This is surprisingly uncommon as tertiary/reparative dentine will often prevent pulpal problems.
- Weakened and chipped incisal edges causing pain from the anterior tip of the tongue (due to the roughness) and poor aesthetics.
- Blue-grey appearance of the thinned enamel incisal edges and possible darkening of teeth due to the change in the optical qualities of the remaining mineralized tissues, again affecting overall aesthetics.

- Loss of tooth structure/fractured teeth or restorations possibly leading to difficulties in chewing due to changes in the occlusion (loss of occlusal contacts, changes in vertical dimension of the bite) and aesthetics.
- Increased risk of marginal fracture of existing restorations as the surrounding hard tissues wear away more rapidly, leaving restorations standing proud.
- Pulpitis, exposure or even loss of vitality attributable to the extent of tissue loss.

Some of these features may need operative treatment to gain immediate relief of acute symptoms or to restore overall dental form and function. However, without the aetiological factor(s) of toothwear being discovered, it will never be cured for that particular patient and the problems will return (see later). Toothwear also needs careful monitoring over a prolonged period to be able to assess its relative progress (see Chapter 8).

2.7 Dental trauma – clinical detection

For patients presenting to general dental practice having sustained facial/oral/dental trauma, it is imperative that before any clinical examination is performed, a thorough history is taken of the incident leading to and causing the trauma. Any suspicions of a head injury including facial fractures (from the history, patient behaviour, general physical examination) should be dealt with by immediate referral to a hospital accident and emergency unit for medical investigation.

Other dentally relevant points to consider are:

- *Patient's age*: stage of tooth/root and soft tissue development and patient compliance issues.
- *Direction of impact/blow/injury*: relevant to the possible direction of displacement of tissues/restorations.
- *Extraoral soft tissue injuries*: examine cheeks, lip lacerations before investigating intraorally. Make clear records with diagrams/photographs (after gaining appropriate consent). Check patient's tetanus status.
- *Teeth*: can the patient occlude their teeth? Have any teeth been avulsed from their sockets – if so, for how long and has the patient

managed to retrieve the tooth? Tooth displacement (including intrusion), mobility (of the individual tooth or dentoalveolar complex), bleeding from intraoral soft tissue wounds. Type of dental fracture sustained (see Figure 2.25).

Note, that if the interval between the injury and presentation is short, pulp vitality testing and percussion tests will have no diagnostic value as the teeth are more than likely to have been concussed and the periodontal ligament bruised. Patient compliance for these investigations (including intraoral radiography) may also be limited! Depending on the severity and symptoms of the injury, it might be worth cleaning up the soft tissue wounds, removing blood clots, debridement under local anaesthesia where necessary and prescribing relevant and necessary antibiotics and pain relief medication at the first visit and then inviting the patient to return after two to three days in order to investigate the dental injuries further and initiate a suitably individualized care plan (see later).

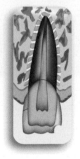 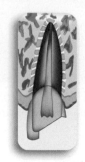 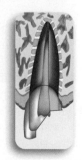 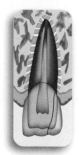 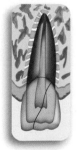 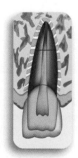

| Enamel infraction Enamel fracture | Enamel + dentine fracture | Enamel + dentine + pulp fracture (complicated fracture) | Uncomplicated crown-root fracture (enamel + dentine + cementum) | Complicated crown-root fracture (e + d + c + pulp) | Root fracture |

Figure 2.25 Classification of traumatic dental tooth fractures. (From Andreasen *et al.* (2007) *Textbook and colour atlas of traumatic injuries to teeth*, 4th edn. Oxford: Blackwell Munksgaard.)

2.8 Developmental defects

As teeth develop and form they are at risk of developing defects that manifest clinically after tooth eruption, often affecting tooth size/shape/number or the quality/quantity of the mineralized tissues themselves. These affected teeth can pose an aesthetic problem and may also be more prone to the ravages of toothwear and/or carious attack. These defects have to be detected and diagnosed from the intraoral dental examination and careful history taking, especially of childhood or maternal illnesses or trauma to the deciduous dentition. Even though developmental defects are relatively rare, the aetiology and clinical appearances of some of the more commonly occurring ones have been described in Table 2.6.

Table 2.6 Developmental defects categorized as acquired and hereditary with their basic aetiology and clinical appearance (in blue) described

Developmental defect		Aetiology/clinical appearance
Acquired	Enamel hypoplasia (Figure 2.26)	Ameloblast damage (systemic childhood infectious diseases, trauma/infection to deciduous predecessor). Hypoplastic – ↓ matrix, normal maturation: **pitted, thin enamel of normal hardness.** Hypomineralized – normal matrix, ↓ mineralization: **opaque, chalky-white, ? softened enamel.** Systemic cause – **defined areas, bands on all teeth developing at time of illness.**
	Molar-incisor hypomineralization (Figure 2.27)	Systemic illness (high fever, respiratory illness) from 0 to 2 years affecting occlusal surfaces of the first molars and possibly maxillary incisors. Hypomineralized – **white-yellow or yellow-brown opacities, easily chipped, ↑ sensitivity (exposed dentine, plaque stagnation).**
	Intrinsic dental fluorosis (Figure 2.28)	Excessive fluoride ion intake (water, toothpaste, tablets) poisons ameloblast function during enamel formation/maturation. **Chalky-white flecks, confluent blotches, brown discoloration, pitted enamel.**
	Intrinsic tetracycline stain (Figure 2.29)	Broad spectrum antibiotic with affinity for mineralized tissues. If taken by mother during pregnancy, deciduous teeth affected; if taken <12 years, permanent teeth affected. Nowadays rare. **Dark, grey horizontal bands affecting all teeth.**
Hereditary (genetic, familial history)	Hypodontia (oligodontia)	Some teeth do not develop; associated with microdontia (**abnormal crown shape/size**). Third molars, second premolars, upper lateral incisors most affected.
	Amelogenesis imperfecta (Figure 2.30)	Abnormalities in enamel formation (complex classification): *Hypoplastic:* defect of matrix formation. **Thin enamel, yellowish teeth (dentine showing through). Or granular, pitted, stained thin enamel.** *Hypomineralized:* defective matrix maturation. **Soft, friable, stained or chalky-white enamel, frequently lost due to weakness at the enamel–dentine junction (EDJ).**
	Dentinogenesis imperfecta	Odontoblast defect affecting dentine matrix formation and mineralization. Rare. **Enamel lost rapidly due to defective EDJ, brown, opalescent dentine colour, prone to fracture/wear. Short roots, bulbous crowns, pulps obliterated.**

2

2

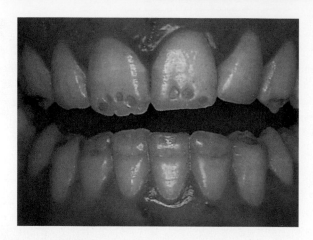

Figure 2.26 Pitted hypoplastic enamel in a patient who experienced a severe childhood illness. Note the pattern of teeth affected – maxillary central incisors and tips of maxillary canines and all mandibular incisors approximately a third of the length from the incisal edges and tips of the mandibular canines too.

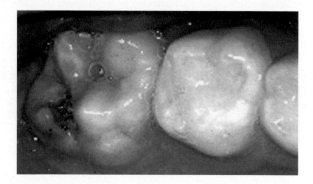

Figure 2.27 Example of molar hypomineralization with yellow-brown opacities on the occlusal surface of UR6. The disto-palatal fissure shows marked enamel breakdown and demarcated border opacities. (Courtesy of K Weerheijm.)

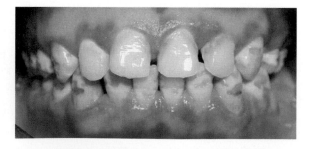

Figure 2.28 Severe dental fluorosis with characteristic generalized enamel pitting and brown discoloration. This patient resided in a Sudanese village with natural fluoride levels in the drinking water exceeding 4000 ppm F. The maxillary central incisors have been polished by a dentist using a fine grit bur, so removing the superficial weakened fluorotic enamel.

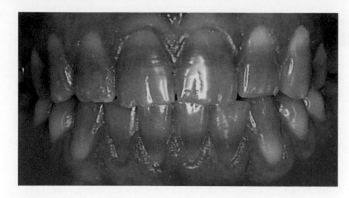

Figure 2.29 Severe intrinsic tetracycline staining with classic horizontal banding of the stain on the labial surfaces.

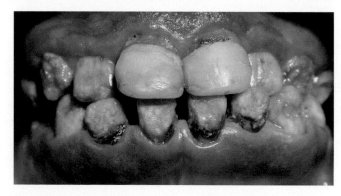

Figure 2.30 Severe hypoplastic amelogenesis imperfecta with hard, thin and pitted enamel remaining on the teeth. The patient presented with two poor quality acrylic crowns on the upper central incisors and buccal cervical caries on the lower incisors.

2.9 Answers to self-test questions

Q2.2: Can you spot an error in the above charting?

A: In the lower left second premolar, there is no MO charted in 'existing restorations' but one has been included in 'treatment to be done'. Well spotted!

Q2.6: What is the name given to the overlying segment of gingivae on the distal aspect of the occlusal surface in both examples above?

A: Gingival operculum.

Q2.7: What hand instrument should be used instead?

A: A blunt, round-headed dental explorer/periodontal probe.

Q2.8: What treatment may be required for this tooth?

A: Initial improvement in oral hygiene to remove the plaque effectively from the occlusal surface. If the patient is not compliant, then an disto-occlusal restoration may be required.

Q2.14: Can you find any more lesions and radiographically classify them? Can you comment on the radiographic changes of the pulp chambers in those teeth?

A: Mesial UR6, distal UR5: D1 – note how even in these relatively distant lesions, tertiary dentine has partly occluded the pulp chambers in these teeth.

Q2.18a: How could you manage this case?

A: Improve oral hygiene and minimally restore the cavity to enable easier biofilm removal.

Q2.19: What stands out as the main problem regarding this patient's sugar intake?

A: The number of episodes per day and their frequency throughout each 24-hour period. This would ensure that the patient's teeth were bathed in plaque with a pH below 5.5 for significant periods leading to demineralization of the enamel.

Q2.21: What would be the obvious cause of the buccal cervical abrasion?

A: Excessive or prolonged action of horizontal toothbrushing.

Q2.22: What might be the presenting complaint of this patient?

A: The appearance of the incisal edges, chipping of the front teeth, sharpness to the tongue, grey discoloration.

Q2.24: What is the cause?

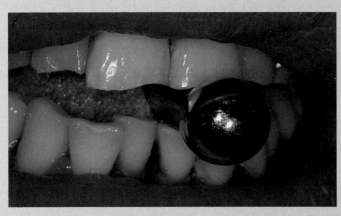

A: The patient plays with a large, metal tongue stud across the anterior teeth causing a significant amount of toothwear damage.

2

3

Diagnosis, prognosis, care planning: 'information processing'

3.1 Introduction

Once a general and targeted history, examination, and other investigations have been carried out (information gathering), it is time for the dentist to assimilate all the relevant information in order to formulate a diagnosis, prognosis, and care plan for the individual patient (information processing). Even though the detection and diagnostic phases have been separated for discussion in this book, an experienced clinician will often accomplish both simultaneously. It is vital to remember that *diagnosis precedes treatment* in all cases.

3.1.1 Definitions

Diagnosis The art or act of inferring from its signs and symptoms or manifestations, the nature or cause of an illness or condition. This stage is critical in order to allow the dentist and the patient to appreciate what is the nature, cause and severity of the condition suffered.

Prognosis The forecast of the course of a disease or the patient's response to treatment of the disease. This stage helps the dentist and patient to understand how easy or difficult the treatment will be to carry out and permit assessment of the patient's motivation to cure the problem. In dentistry, the dental team can only start the patient off on the road to recovery by restoring form and function to their dentition as well as helping the patient to prevent/control the disease process so preventing its return. It is then up to the patient as to whether they follow this advice and maintain their oral health in the future.

Care plan (treatment plan) The formal itemized management strategy developed for the individual patient to treat the manifestations of an illness and to control/prevent the illness from reoccurring. This can be divided into phases of therapy (e.g. prevention/control, stabilization, definitive treatment, monitoring), should be adapted and modified during its execution for maximum benefit to the patient. It should take into account unforeseen developments in the course of the disease or the patient's response to care. It should be written and made clear to all parties for discussion so that informed consent can be gained prior to implementation.

3.2 Diagnosing dental pain, 'toothache'

Common diseases occur commonly. A list of common diagnoses of dental pain is given below and the various features of each are summarized in Table 3.2:

- Acute pulpitis
- Acute periapical periodontitis
- Acute periapical abscess
- Acute periodontal (lateral) abscess
- Chronic pulpitis
- Chronic periapical periodontitis (apical granuloma)
- Exposed sensitive dentine
- Interproximal food-packing
- Cracked cusps/tooth syndrome

Other conditions outwith the remit of this book may also manifest as dentofacial pain: maxillary sinusitis, trigeminal neuralgia, facial arthromyalgia, pericoronitis. It must be understood that pain symptoms rarely fall neatly into the diagnoses listed above (see also Table 3.2) and that a degree of clinical experience will be required to interpret the relevant signs and symptoms to permit a diagnosis to be made. It is important to recognize that the signs and symptoms from an inflamed pulp do not necessarily correlate with the histological changes that are occurring within that pulp. Therefore, interpretation of the signs and symptoms must be carried out with caution.

3.2.1 Acute pulpitis

- Acute, severe, poorly localized pain.
- Does not cross the facial midline and might be difficult for patients to identify from which jaw it is originating. They may present holding their face on the relevant side, rather than identifying a particular tooth.
- There are two clinical presentations (not necessarily relating to pulpal histology), *reversible* and *irreversible*. Table 3.1 highlights their similarities and differences.
- Clinically, offending teeth may present with carious lesions or large restorations which may be defective, but the dentist must always check the status of the dentition in both quadrants on the relevant side.

3.2.2 Acute periapical periodontitis

- Pain localizable to the offending tooth – patient will be able to point to it and will complain of pain on biting onto it (due to stimulation of pain and pressure-sensitive fibres in the periodontal ligament).
- Tooth tender to palpate/percussion (if the patient permits this!).
- Tenderness felt over the root apex through mucosae in the buccal sulcus.
- Pulp may initially retain vitality but will eventually become necrotic.
- Periapical radiograph *may* show loss of lamina dura around the root apex region during late stage presentation.

3.2.3 Acute periapical abscess

- Patient may present with a large facial/intraoral swelling associated with the affected relevant quadrant or a more localized swelling in the alveolar mucosa over the affected root.
- May present before swelling occurs or after it has burst and subsided, with evidence of a sinus tract.

Table 3.1 Characteristics of acute pulpitis

Reversible pulpitis	Irreversible pulpitis
Characteristic short, sharp pain	Characteristic dull, throbbing pain (but may experience bouts of sharp pain)
Stimulated by hot, cold or sweet stimuli	Onset usually unprovoked/**exacerbated** by hot, cold, sweet stimuli
Few seconds duration/**disappears** when stimulus removed	**Several minutes/hours** duration/**persists** when stimulus removed
Pulp sensibility tests may elicit an exaggerated response	Pulp sensibility tests may elicit an exaggerated/negative response
Tooth not tender to percussion (TTP)	Tooth not TTP (unless late stage presentation)

- Patient may present with fever.
- Tooth will be painful to bite on, negative results with vitality tests (if permitted).
- Periapical radiograph will usually show loss of lamina dura and widening of the periodontal ligament space around the root apex.

3.2.4 Acute periodontal (lateral) abscess

- Forms at the base of a deep periodontal pocket.
- Well-localized pain that is associated with a vital pulp.
- If this is combined with pulpal necrosis (of differing aetiology) then a 'perio-endo' lesion can be diagnosed, often with poor prognosis, leading to extraction of the tooth.

3.2.5 Chronic pulpitis

- Mild, poorly localized, periodic grumbling pain (on and off) over several weeks/months.
- Initially vital pulp and tooth not TTP but if condition progresses, eventually symptoms of periapical periodontitis may supervene.
- Initial treatment will be monitoring to assess whether the pulp has recovered after treating the cause, e.g. caries, cracked tooth.
- More severe cases will require removal of any restoration, placement of a sedative dressing over the pulp, and then a provisional restoration.

3.2.6 Chronic periapical periodontitis

- Can be symptomless or elicit mild pain on biting
- Positive response to vigorous percussion or even presentation with a sinus tract (see Figure 3.2 below).
- Periapical radiograph shows well demarcated radiolucency around the root apex (see Figure 3.1)
- Often described as an apical granuloma.

- The apical granuloma is a chronic inflammatory response (highly vascularized granulation tissue) to toxins leaching from the necrotic pulp causing increased osteoclastic action in the subjacent bone leading to bone resorption. As the toxins dilute, the extent of the resorption is naturally limited. If the necrotic pulp, and therefore the source of toxins, is removed bony repair can result (see Figure 3.1).
- If infection occurs, the chronic apical granuloma can flare up into an acute apical abscess with sinus tract (see Figure 3.2).
- Chronic apical granulomas may become cystic and require surgical intervention for treatment (see Figure 3.3).

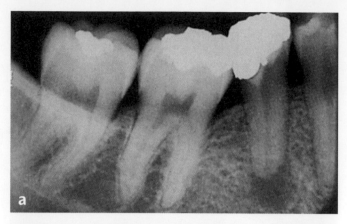
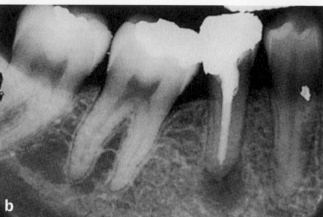
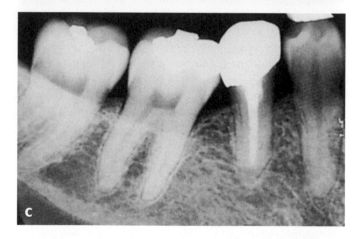

Figure 3.1 (a) Periapical radiograph showing a well-demarcated radiolucency at the apex of LR5 (with accompanying loss of lamina dura and relative widening of the periodontal ligament space when compared with the adjacent healthy LR7). The large restoration has contributed to pulp necrosis in this tooth and it is likely that a periapical granuloma has formed, but this should strictly be diagnosed from histological analysis of a biopsy sample. (b) Periapical radiograph of the same tooth after the gutta percha root filling was placed. (c) Radiograph three years later showing healing around the root apex of the LR5, bony infill and re-formed lamina dura. (Courtesy of late Professor Pitt Ford.)

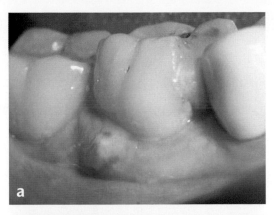

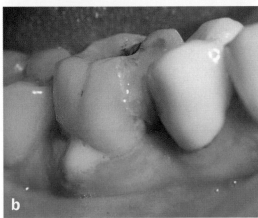

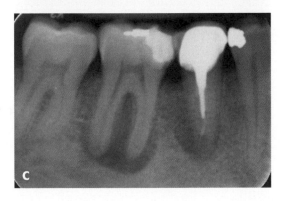

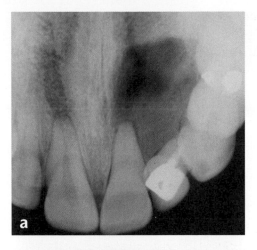

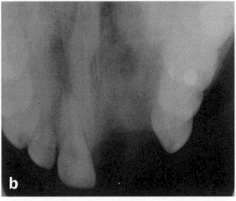

Figure 3.3 (**a**) Upper standard occlusal radiographs showing large palatal cystic change in an apical granuloma associated with UL12. (**b**) Same radiograph taken three years later after UL12 were extracted and the cyst surgically managed. Note the near complete bony infill of the initially large defect. Implants were successfully placed into the new bone to restore UL12.

Figure 3.2 Chronically infected apical granuloma (**a**) with pus pointing through a sinus on the mucosa adjacent to the non-vital LR6 (**b**). (**c**) Periapical radiograph shows a large radiolucency associated with the apices and furcation of the LR6 as well as a separate periapical radiolucency on the heavily restored (but inadequately root-treated) LR5.

- To reduce the sensitivity, the exposed tubules may be blocked using a dentine bonding agent or thin layer of resin composite. Use of potassium nitrate/chloride compounds may help to reduce tubule conduction and pain transmission. Treatments involving bioactive glasses are showing promise in reducing sensitivity.

3.2.8 Interproximal food-packing

- Open contact point (drifted teeth, poor contouring of adjacent proximal restorations) enables food debris to get caught between teeth and traumatize the interdental periodontal papillae leading to localized tenderness, bleeding, and inflammation.

3.2.9 Cracked cusp/tooth syndrome

- Cracks can involve enamel only (no pain – similar to superficial cracks in a porcelain teacup) or enamel and dentine (± pulp), which can cause poorly localized pain periodically.

- There is sometimes a sharp pain on biting/thermal stimulus. Pulp tests may be inconclusive, as well as percussion/palpation tests.

3.2.7 Exposed sensitive dentine

- Poorly localized short, sharp sensitivity to hot, cold, or sweet stimuli caused by exposed root dentine surfaces (gingival recession, root caries). The pain response can be elicited by air-drying the exposed surface using a dental 3-1 air/water syringe.

- Positive pulp test (perhaps slightly hyper-responsive if tested during an acute episode), teeth not TTP.

Table 3.2 Classic signs and symptoms for differential diagnoses for dental pain. Unfortunately, not all symptoms fall into these clear categories and experience is required for their interpretation

	Acute pulpitis	Acute apical periodontitis	Acute apical abscess	Acute periodontal abscess	Exposed sensitive dentine	Food packing	Cracked cusp	Chronic pulpitis	Chronic apical periodontitis (apical granuloma)
History	Recent pain with hot and cold. May be very severe. Poorly localized.	Tender to bite. Well localized.	Pain and swelling. Very well localized.	Localized swelling. Some pain.	Generalized pain to hot and cold, and sweet.	Pain after eating fibrous food, e.g. meat.	Vague intermittent pain usually on biting. May be poorly localized.	Vague, unprovoked intermittent but increasing pain. Poorly localized.	May have had pain in the past. Now not sensitive to hot and cold.
Clinical examination	Possibly caries or recent large restoration.	Possibly caries.	May be extraoral or intraoral swelling over apex of tooth.	Intraoral swelling nearer to gingival margin. Tooth may be mobile.	Gingival recession. Exposed dentine at the gingival margin. Sensitive to probe or cold air.	Open contact points. Gingival inflammation. Food usually present.	Often nothing, but crack may be seen. May be painful with occlusal contact *only*.	May have large restoration or caries.	May have large restoration or caries.
Vitality test	Hypersensitive.	May still be vital, but usually non-vital.	Non-vital.	Often vital.	Vital.	May be vital or non-vital.	May be hypersensitive.	Often normal but may be hypersensitive.	Non-vital.
Percussion	Not tender.	Tender.	Tender to touch. Too tender to percuss.	Slight tenderness, more to lateral than axial pressure.	Not tender.	Not tender to percussion. May be sore with lateral percussion.	Usually not tender but may be.	Not tender.	Slightly. May give dull sound on percussion.
Other clinical tests			Raised temperature. Looks ill.	Deep pockets. Pus may be released on probing pocket.		Floss passes the contact easily.	Sometimes tender to lateral pressure on an individual cusp.		
Radiographic findings	Probably caries close to pulp. No periapical change.	Usually no periapical change in early stage.	Usually no periapical change except slight thickening of apical periodontal membrane.	Alveolar bone loss. Usually no periapical change.	May be some alveolar bone loss.	None.	None.	None.	Periapical radiolucency.
Findings on further investigations	Carious exposure of pulp.	Necrotic pulp.	Pus may be drained via abscess cavity to root canal without local anaesthetic, giving immediate relief of pain and confirming the diagnosis.				Crack sometimes visible at base of cavity when old restoration removed. If left, cuspal fracture will eventually occur.	Symptoms may settle if restoration removed and tooth dressed with calcium hydroxide, but pulp often dies eventually.	Necrotic pulp.

3

- Transillumination or dyes can be used to detect cracks, but do not relate their presence to cause of pain.
- Diagnostic test may involve careful analysis of pain on biting. Using a cotton wool roll, wood stick (wooden tongue depressor split lengthways), rubber suction tip or proprietary kits, e.g. Tooth Sleuth, cracked tooth/cusp pain can be elicited on specific cusps, at specific angles of pressure and assessed on biting and release. This helps to ascertain where and how deep the crack might be and therefore what treatment is required.

3.3 Caries risk/susceptibility assessment

The aetiology, histopathology, and detection methods for caries have been discussed in Chapters 1 and 2. Once this information has been gathered through a targeted verbal history and examination, analysis ('information processing') is required to ascertain the risk potential of the individual patient to developing further disease and responding to treatment of current disease. This is known as a caries risk/susceptibility assessment.

Table 3.3 Factors involved in assessing caries risk and categorizing the patient's susceptibility to caries as high or low risk*

Caries risk assessment		
High risk		**Low risk**
Social history	Socially deprived High caries in siblings Low knowledge of dental disease Irregular attender Ready availability of snacks Low dental aspirations	Middle class Low caries in siblings Dentally aware Regular attender Work does not allow regular snacks High dental aspirations
Medical history	Medically compromised Disabled Xerostomia Long-term cariogenic medicine	No medical problem No physical problem Normal salivary flow No long-term medication
Dietary habits	Frequent sugar intake	Infrequent sugar intake
Fluoride use	Non-fluoride area No fluoride supplements No fluoride toothpaste	Fluoridation area Fluoride supplements used Fluoride toothpaste used
Plaque control	Infrequent, ineffective, cleaning Poor manual control	Frequent/effective cleaning Good manual control
Saliva	Low flow rate Low buffering capacity High *Streptococcus mutans* and Lactobacillus counts	Normal flow rate High buffering capacity Low *S. mutans* and lactobacillus counts
Clinical evidence	New lesions Premature extractions Anterior caries or restorations Multiple restorations History of repeated restorations No fissure sealants Multiband orthodontics Partial dentures	No new lesions Nil extractions for caries Sound anterior teeth No or few restorations Restorations inserted years ago Fissure sealed No appliances

*This information can be gathered from a targeted verbal history and examination (Chapter 2).

3

Table 3.4 An example chart to note down key findings from the patient's history/examination in order to help evaluate their caries risk

Status	'Yes' answer: High risk	'No' answer: Low risk
Lesions: ≥2 new/progressing/restored lesions in the last two years?		
General factors		
Diet: Frequent snacks between meals? Anorexia, bulimia?		
Fluoride: No fluoride (toothpaste/rinse daily, fluoridated water community)?		
Health: Sjögren's syndrome, chemotherapy, radiation to head and neck?		
Medications: Hypo-salivatory medication?		
Social: Low socioeconomic status? Parents/siblings with active caries?		
Age: Adolescent? Elderly?		
Oral factors		
OH: Quality? What aids are used?		
Saliva: Stimulated saliva flow <0.7ml/min?		
Plaque: Readily visible heavy plaque – plaque scores?		
Bacterial balance: Levels of *S. mutans*.		

Adapted from Domejean *et al.* Minimal Intervention Treatment Plan (MITP): practical implementation in general practice. *J Min Intervent Dent* 2009;**2**:103–23.

3

Without this knowledge, caries management at the individual patient level will never be successful in the long term. Risk assessments can also be carried out at a population level in order to help promote prevention strategies for large numbers of people, e.g. water fluoridation programmes.

- It makes economic sense to target preventive treatments in practice at the appropriate risk group.
- Dental care neither begins nor ends with a single course of treatment but is ongoing. When a course of dental treatment is complete, the dentist and patient decide when it would be wise to check that all is well. This recall interval is based partly on an assessment of the risk of disease progression and should not be standardized at six months or any other period.
- Patients should be made aware of their risk status. This knowledge encourages them to keep appropriate recall appointments, to become *motivated* and involved in their own preventive care, and, if they pay for their treatment, it may help them budget for dental bills.

The various patient factors that affect the risk assessment have been highlighted in Table 3.3. The relevance of these factors in a targeted verbal history of risk assessment have been included in Table 2.1 (Chapter 2) and a chart similar to Table 3.4 might be used in the patient notes to document such findings. The caries risk assessment will change over time and therefore should be assessed when the pattern of disease presentation changes in the same patient: the overall management of caries is as dynamic as the disease process itself.

In terms of the numbers of lesions detected during the clinical oral examination, a high caries risk patient is one who presents with, or has a past history of ≥2 new/progressing/restored carious lesions in the previous two years. The patient's caries risk can be classified into three categories, low, medium or high, but with relevance to clinical dental practice management, a simpler division into low or high risk/susceptibility is usually sufficient and helps to structure their individualized care plan accordingly (see later).

3.4 Diagnosing toothwear

The detection and diagnosis of toothwear from its causative factors has been discussed in detail in Chapter 2. A targeted verbal history coupled with rigorous examination of the teeth is essential to return a diagnosis of this common multifactorial problem. Differentiating between acceptable age-related and pathological levels of wear can be difficult as this depends on the patient's age, dental history, and the rate of progress of the toothwear, which can be clinically difficult to assess unless the patient is reviewed annually in the first instance. However, wear facets with staining present may be indicative of a very slow or arrested rate of progress, whereas significant dental sensitivity from such lesions may indicate a more rapid rate of wear, as there would not have been enough time for the upregulated odontoblasts to lay down translucent or tertiary dentine (see Chapter 1 – *Dentine–pulp complex reparative reactions*).

3.5 Diagnosing dental trauma and developmental defects

Again, as with toothwear above, the degree of separation between detection and diagnosis of trauma and developmental defects is negligible as the two processes are intimately linked with the verbal history and the oral/dental examination. These have been discussed in detail in Chapter 2.

3.6 Prognostic indicators

A dentist should give the patient a verbal and written prognosis for the individual tooth/teeth requiring interventional treatment and/or a prognosis for the treatment of the overall condition the patient has. At the tooth level, factors affecting the prognosis include:

- The severity of damage incurred to the coronal hard tissues (extent of the carious lesion, amount of tooth structure lost due to trauma/toothwear/developmental defect). Can operative treatment repair and reinstate the tooth structure successfully in the mid-long term?
- The status of the pulp
- The status of the periodontium (alveolar bone levels, periodontal ligament).

In terms of the underlying condition, prognostic factors include:

- The ease with which the aetiological factors can be removed/modified to prevent or slow the progress of the disease and its reoccurrence. As an example, the aetiology of xerostomia caused by radiation therapy cannot be modified so dental conditions (caries) will generally have a poor prognosis. However, with very good oral hygiene procedures and the use of fluoride, the prognosis might be slightly improved.
- The overall level of patient motivation to manage the condition. If a patient is not particularly concerned then the long-term outlook for treatment will be bleak at best, and only repairs may be considered.

3.7 Formulating an individualized care plan (treatment plan)

3.7.1 Why is a care plan necessary?

The need and importance of making individualized, adaptable plans, both simple and complex, and of recording the decisions in the patient's record can be summarized as follows:

- It ensures that the lead clinician reviews the treatment in the light of all available evidence at the start of treatment and at stages throughout it.
- It is a record for later reference, particularly in complicated cases and after a lapse of time. This is available mostly for the benefit of the patient, but on occasions, when patients complain, it may have dento-legal importance and may protect the dentist against unjustified complaints. In this context, when the treatment plan is complex and expensive, it may be wise to put the advice in the form of a letter to the patient so that he or she has time to consider it and its implications before acceptance or rejection. The letter is also a written record, of which the patient has a copy, in cases where there is a dento-legal problem later.
- It avoids the risk of disordered and ill-advised treatment, which may arise if treatment is undertaken piecemeal.

Written care plans however simple, should be made for every patient. Written care plans should be specifically tailored to each patient's needs, and taking all factors into consideration from the detection and diagnostic phases, must have realistic goals and be achievable for both the dentist and the patient.

Patients must understand the implications of the treatment and appreciate thatp the care plan may deviate from the initial path as required. They must also appreciate their own role in its ultimate success, the timeframe for its delivery, and its cost (if applicable).

3.7.2 Structure of a care plan

However simple a care plan may be for a particular management episode, it is wise to have a structure to follow. One such scheme is outlined in Table 3.5:

- An initial *stabilization phase* (which may take several months to complete depending on the amount/type of work required).
- Followed by *reassessment* – to re-evaluate the response to initial treatment and the future needs of the patient.
- A *rehabilitation phase* – where definitive restorations can be designed and placed.

Other considerations include the type of restorative material to use (see Chapter 6) and whether operative intervention will be minimal, or whether it will be more extensive (i.e. whether to restore or attempt to arrest a carious lesion in dentine/restore or monitor an erosive toothwear lesion/extract or endodontically treat an infected tooth).

Table 3.5 A care plan flowchart structuring the treatment into three phases, which can blend into one another depending on the complexity of the plan

Care plan phases	Comments
Stabilization	Pain relief ↓ Control active disease Prevention Extraction of teeth with hopeless prognosis Transitional restorations ↓
Reassess	Reassess patients' response to the stabilization phase, their subsequent needs, aesthetic expectations, motivation, dental examination, costs ↓
Rehabilitation	Reorganizing or conforming to existing occlusal scheme (see later); definitive restorations/prostheses ↓ Review and maintenance

These decisions must be made with input from the patient (including their own perceived need, aesthetic considerations, number of appointments, costs, dental anxiety) as this will confer some ownership and therefore responsibility to the patient in terms of the success of the final outcome. Second opinions from more experienced specialists in practice or hospital can be very helpful especially for the more complex cases, especially as there is rarely an absolute right or wrong decision made in care planning. Choosing the best option from several for the patient is a skill that comes with further clinical experience, and unfortunately, making some errors in judgement along the way! It is vital to learn from these situations and adapt accordingly in the future.

Table 4.1 (Chapter 4) gives an example of a care plan flowchart for patients with dental caries. It is based on five possible management options dependent on the presence/absence of lesions coupled with the individual's caries risk assessment. Of course, real life is not always that simple and patients' conditions do not always fit into such clear-cut categories, but this concept mapping helps the dentist and the patient understand the options and where the management strategy chosen fits in, with respect to the alternatives.

4
Disease control and lesion prevention

Chapter contents

4.1 Introduction

From the previous chapter it can be seen that in all cases of caries and toothwear, disease control and lesion prevention are key aspects of the management strategy, often commencing in the stabilization phase of the care plan but continuing throughout the full course of treatment.

Disease control Neither the dentist nor the patient has the power to *prevent* the carious or toothwear process. These ubiquitous processes occur at the ionic, metabolic, and microscopic level at the tooth surface/biofilm interface and are made pathological by other factors. However, if these factors are controlled/modified, then the process can be also.

Lesion prevention The term prevention has commonly been used to describe the above, but actually it is only the manifestation of the pathological process, i.e. the lesion in caries or toothwear, that can be *prevented* if the disease process is controlled.

4.2 Caries control (and lesion prevention)

4.2.1 Categorizing caries activity and risk status

On the basis of the history and examination, the patient may be allocated to one of the following in terms of caries activity/risk status:

- *Caries inactive/caries controlled/low risk*: no active lesions and no history of recurrent restorations in the past two to three years. A level of control is still required to remain in this stable condition.
- *Caries active/modifiable risk factors/high risk* (plaque control, fluoride, diet): presence of active lesions and a yearly increment of

4

more than two new/progressing/filled lesions in the preceding two to three years. Caries control may be achieved by changing risk factors.

- *Caries active/unmodifiable or unidentifiable risk factors/high risk* (dry mouths, medications): this category will always be high risk although it may still be possible to control caries by optimal control of risk factors. Presence of active lesions and a yearly increment of more than two new/progressing/filled lesions in the preceding two to three years.

The aim is to help the patient change the risk factors so that at recall, the caries activity status may be deemed to have changed because there are no new active lesions and/or lesions previously judged as active are now deemed arrested. Table 4.1 shows a flowchart of potential care plans depending on lesion presence (activity) and the patient's caries risk. Note in all cases, disease control is paramount in preventing further lesion development, but there are different levels of control that can be offered depending on the activity/risk status: *standard* and *active* care (Table 4.2).

4.2.2 Standard care (non-operative, preventive therapy) – low risk, caries-controlled patient

The standard care regimen is carried out wholly by the patient on the advice of the dental care professional.

Plaque control

Caries lesions form as a result of the metabolic events in dental plaque. Thus plaque control is the logical cornerstone of non-operative treatment. Teeth should be brushed with a fluoride-containing toothpaste as it interferes with growth and ecology of the biofilm and fluoride application retards lesion progression.

Table 4.1 A care plan flowchart for caries management showing the interaction of caries susceptibility, presence/absence of lesions, and an emphasis on minimally invasive dentistry for the operative treatment of individual lesions with suitable recall intervals

Identify (Chapter 2)	Lesion			No lesion	
	Cavitated (Irreversible)	Non-cavitated (Reversible)			
Caries susceptibility	High/low caries risk 3, 4 (mICDAS)	High risk 0, 1, 2	Low risk 0, 1, 2	High risk	Low risk
Control (prevent) (Chapter 4) Preventive treatment and patient motivation	**SC + Active care plus:** Pit and fissure sealants Patient motivation	**SC + Active care:** Remin Fluoride CPP-ACP PMTC Patient motivation	**SC + Active care:** Remin Fluoride CPP-ACP PMTC Patient motivation	**SC + Active care:** Fluoride CPP-ACP PMTC Patient motivation	**Standard care (SC)/ maintenance** Oral hygiene Diet control Fluoride toothpaste
Restore (Chapter 7)	Transitional restorations: GIC Long-term restorations: GIC/ composites	Preventive resin restorations	–	–	–
Recall (Chapter 8)	2–6 months	3–6 months	6–12 months	3–6 months	12–18 months

*The column on the left indicates where in this book those topics are discussed in detail.
See Table 4.2 for explanations of standard care and active care regimens.
CPP-ACP, casein phosphopeptide – amorphous calcium phosphate; PMTC, professional mechanical tooth cleaning.
Adapted from Domejean *et al*. Minimal Intervention Treatment Plan (MITP): practical implementation in general practice. *J Min Intervent Dent* 2009;**2**:103–23.

The preventive action of tooth brushing can be maximized if the following principles are followed.

- Brushing should start as soon as the first deciduous tooth erupts.
- Brush twice daily, last thing at night and at one other time each day.
- Discourage rinsing with lots of water after brushing; 'spit, don't rinse' is the relevant advice.
- Children under 3 years should use a toothpaste containing no less than 1000 ppm (parts per million) fluoride.
- Children between 3 and 6 years are likely to swallow toothpaste and this may cause fluorosis. To prevent this they should use only a smear of paste (pea-sized amount) and not be allowed to eat or lick toothpaste from the tube.
- Currently, it is recommended that over the age of 3 years, family fluoride toothpaste (1350–1500 ppm fluoride) should be used.
- Children need to be helped and supervised by an adult when brushing.
- The occlusal surface of erupting molars should be individually brushed with the brush placed at right angles to the arch.
- Dependant adults should be helped with tooth cleaning.

Oral hygiene instruction (OHI) should be general to the whole mouth and site-specific to the particular lesion. The patient should be aware of the problem areas, seeing these in their mouths (via mirrors/intraoral cameras) and/or on a radiograph. The following may be helpful with respect to tooth brushing:

- The patient should attend each appointment with their brush and toothpaste.
- Check the toothpaste for fluoride content and the brush head quality to ensure it is not worn.
- Disclose the mouth with a suitable plaque-staining dye so that this can be clearly seen by the patient.
- Assess whether the patient (or parent/carer) can remove the plaque or should the technique/brush be altered? Arthritic patients, for example, may not be able to manipulate the normal handle of a toothbrush so silicone impression material or cold-cure acrylic may be used to thicken the grip to aid manual dexterity. Electric toothbrushes may also be recommended.
- Is thorough brushing in the surgery causing gingival bleeding? If so, does the patient realize this indicates gingivitis caused by dental plaque?
- If active lesions are present, is the patient aware where they are and able to remove disclosed plaque from them?

Where active approximal lesions are present, either in the enamel or on the root surface, an interdental cleaning aid will be needed. In young patients, lesions are best cleaned with floss, whereas interdental brushes are preferred for cleaning larger interdental spaces following gingival recession. The following may be helpful with respect to interdental cleaning:

- Advice given must be site-specific.
- Examining the tape or brush after use may show the plaque that has been removed and this can be a useful motivating factor.
- A special holder for the floss or brush may help the patient.

- Super-floss may be used to clean around bridge pontics or crown margins.
- If the gingivae bleed, the relevance of this should be explained to the patient. If bleeding persists for days after effective cleaning is instituted, this may indicate a cavity or plaque-retentive feature is present that prevents the patient removing the plaque. A restoration may be needed to restore tooth integrity to allow the surface to be cleaned.

Use of fluoride

Fluoride delays lesion progression by being physico-chemically incorporated into the hydroxyapatite lattice structure and by inhibiting carbohydrate metabolism within the plaque bacteria (enolase and phosphoenolpyruvate (PEP)-phosphotransferase system inhibition). Vehicles for fluoride include:

- Water – to date, only approximately 15% of the UK population has access to 1 ppm F$^-$ water.
- Toothpaste – fluoride toothpaste is cheap, requires minimal patient cooperation, and enhances patients' appreciation of their essential role in caries control. See above for advice on fluoride concentration and toothpaste use.

The choice of vehicle is not crucial, but it must be combined with improvement in oral hygiene. It is important that the patient accepts the mode of treatment and complies with advice.

Dietary modification

The evidence that the frequency and amount of sugar consumption is linked to caries is irrefutable. Thus emphasis on diet in caries control would seem logical. Unfortunately, the evidence that it is possible to modify people's diets is lacking! Since the advent of fluoride, the emphasis in caries control has shifted from diet to oral hygiene with a fluoride-containing toothpaste. However, this does not preclude the dental professional from giving dietary advice to all patients. Reducing the amount and frequency of sugary food intake can reduce dental caries and could help weight control. All health professionals have a responsibility to give advice on diet, in the same way as they have a responsibility to give advice on smoking cessation.

No change in diet should be advised for the caries-inactive/controlled patient, but the dentist should make the patient aware of how an adverse change in diet and/or salivary flow could pose a problem, especially if oral hygiene is poor. All patients should be aware of the link between sugar and caries.

All of the above aspects of *standard care* for controlling disease and preventing lesions require patient cooperation and motivation. The dental team is the adviser and the patients the executors of their own preventive care plan.

4.2.3 Active care – high risk/uncontrolled patient

This regimen includes all aspects of standard care *plus* those listed in Table 4.2, where the dental team may have to take on some of the treatment as well as an advisory role.

Table 4.2 Features of preventive treatment regimens, standard and active care, to control caries and prevent lesions developing or progressing

Standard care (patient-led, non-operative) Inactive/controlled, low risk patient	Active care (dentist-led, operative/non-operative) Active/uncontrolled, high risk patient
Plaque control (toothbrush and toothpaste, flossing) Use of **fluoride** (toothpaste, water) **Dietary** modification **Patient motivation** paramount to prevent onset of disease	STANDARD CARE +: **Decontamination** procedures (PMTC, transitional restorations, chlorhexidine) **Remineralization** procedures: • Fluoride (high concentration toothpaste, mouthwashes, topical varnishes) • Remineralizing pastes/solutions (e.g. CPP-ACP) **Managing hyposalivation** (medications, saliva substitutes) **Fissure sealant restorations**

Decontamination procedures

Professional mechanical tooth cleaning (PMTC) This is carried out by members of the dental team (dentist, hygienist, therapist) using hand scalers/ultrasonic/air-polishing instrumentation to remove gross calculus deposits, and rotating brushes with prophy paste to debride mechanically particularly thick, tenacious plaque deposits on the tooth surfaces. This will then allow the patient to clean more effectively with their toothbrush whilst enabling the clinician to examine the tooth surfaces directly.

Transitional (stabilizing) restorations In some cases (e.g. rampant caries) early stabilizing adhesive restorations (glass ionomer cements (GICs)/resin modified (RM)-GICs – see Chapters 6 and 7) can be placed, not only to strengthen remaining tooth structure but also to remove the carious biomass, which acts as a bacterial reservoir and is impossible to clean effectively with conventional oral hygiene procedures (see Figure 4.1).

Chlorhexidine (CHX) rinses There is little clinical evidence for the use of chlorhexidine in the medium- to long-term control of caries. CHX (>0.12%) can affect plaque biofilm adherence and bacterial diversity on a short-term basis and can be used post oral surgical procedures when normal oral hygiene procedures would be difficult to perform due to pain, risk of postoperative bleeding, and swelling. Long-term use may lead to altered taste perception, extrinsic dental staining, and possible mucosal irritation, and is therefore not recommended.

Remineralization procedures
Fluoride

• High concentration prescription toothpastes can be beneficial to control caries (2800/5000 ppm fluoride) for high risk patients (multiple lesions, dry mouth).

• Fluoride mouthwash can be prescribed for patients aged ≥8 years, for daily (0.05% NaF)/weekly (0.2% NaF) use. Below 8 years, these mouthwashes are not advised because there is a risk of sufficient mouthwash to cause fluorosis in the developing dentition.

The rinse should be in addition to twice-daily brushing with toothpaste containing at least 1350 ppm fluoride. Rinses require patient compliance and should be used at a different time to tooth brushing to maximize the topical effect, which relates to frequency of availability. The product should be rinsed around the mouth for a timed minute. Be aware that some products are astringent and will be uncomfortable for children and painful for those with a dry mouth. A bland, non-alcoholic mouthwash should be advised. The indications for the use of fluoride mouthwash are:

– Patients over 8 years with high caries activity.

– Patients with orthodontic appliances, which inevitably encourage plaque accumulation and predispose to carious lesions.

– Patients with a dry mouth (xerostomia).

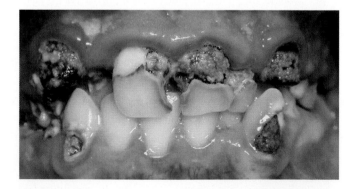

Figure 4.1 An anterior view of a 24-year-old caries-active/uncontrolled, high risk patient with rampant caries. The large cavitated lesions are covered with a tenacious plaque biofilm. In such patients, transitional (stabilizing) restorations might be necessary to remove the bacterial reservoir and to recontour the smooth tooth/restoration surfaces to facilitate improved oral hygiene procedures.

Q4.1: What might be the possible aetiology of this degree of caries attack?

– Patients developing root caries. In these patients a weekly concentrated mouthwash may be advised for daily use.

• Professionally applied fluoride varnishes/fluids (e.g. Duraphat, Elmex Fluid) with concentrations of 22 600 ppm F or 2.2% F. Systematic reviews of research have shown fluoride varnish application by dental care professionals can reduce caries increment in the deciduous dentition by a third and by nearly half in the permanent dentition. These are impressive reductions in caries, but the dental professional should be aware that:

– Professional application must be repeated at 3-monthly (high risk child/adult) to 6-monthly (3 years to teens, adults with dry mouth/active caries) intervals to be effective and this is inevitably costly.

– The emphasis switches to the care being by the professional rather than by the patient.

– The concentration of fluoride is high and this means the varnish is potentially toxic to a small child if swallowed. The maximum dose advised for use in the primary dentition is 0.25 ml and in the mixed dentition is 0.5 ml.

– The varnish should be applied to isolated, clean, dry teeth. An ideal time to apply varnish is therefore when the teeth are being examined for carious lesions because to detect lesions, the teeth must be isolated, clean, and dry (see Chapter 2). Once the charting is complete, it takes only seconds to apply varnish to fissures, over contact points, cervical margins buccally and lingually, and exposed root surfaces.

Topical remineralizing agents Research is being carried out into the development of calcium and phosphate-rich ionic solutions or pastes that can potentially act as a reservoir for these mineralizing ions so encouraging surface remineralization. CPP-ACP (casein phosphopeptide – amorphous calcium phosphate $(Ca_9(PO_4)_6 + H_2O))$ is one such product, sold under the trade name Recaldent. ACP has a natural predilection to convert to hydroxyapatite (HAP) in wet, ionically favourable environments, and the phosphopeptide chains are thought to help bind these complexes to the tooth/biofilm surfaces and envelop them, so regulating and directing the ultimate precipitation of the HAP where it is needed, i.e. demineralized surfaces. Combinations of CCP-ACP with fluoride have also been developed and clinical evidence is being gathered as to their overall efficacy in preventive management of early carious and fluorotic lesions, especially in adults where the mix of fluoride, calcium, and phosphate ions seem to have a synergistic effect (see Figure 4.2). Current evidence tends towards a favourable short-term remineralizing effect, but further long-term trials are needed.

Managing hyposalivation

Controlling caries when the mouth is dry is very difficult. A dry mouth is miserable for the patient and can be a worry for the dentist. The management approach for caries control in these high risk patients should be:

• Immaculate oral hygiene.

• Prescribe a high fluoride toothpaste (5000 ppm F).

• Prescribe a fluoride mouthwash (non-alcohol containing).

• Apply fluoride varnish to lesions every 3 months (see above).

• Ask the patient to keep a diet sheet and try to minimize sugar intake.

• Be aware that the patient needs to moisten their mouth frequently and that plain water is safe.

• Recall the patient every 3 months.

• Saliva may be stimulated by chewing a xylitol-containing chewing gum, provided there is sufficient salivary gland activity or pharmacologically.

• In cases of Sjögren's syndrome or post radiotherapy, a saliva substitute may be required.

• Check that any prescribed antifungal agent does not contain sugar.

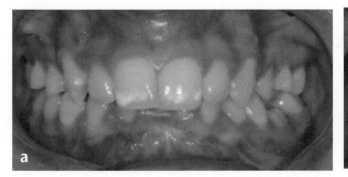
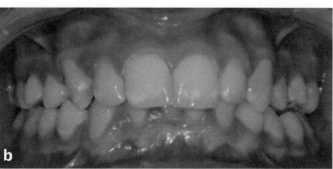

Figure 4.2 (a) Patient with chalky, matt fluorotic lesions on the labial surfaces of the upper central incisors (see Chapter 2, Table 2.6). **(b)** One month later, after professional application of topical fluoride/CPP-ACP paste. The lesions are not as clinically evident. (Courtesy of Dr M Basso.)

Q4.2: How can you distinguish these lesions from white spot carious lesions?

4

● Check with the medical practitioner regarding alternatives to medications causing hyposalivation (this may be limited as the medical benefits of the medication will usually outweigh the negative effect of the reduced saliva output).

Fissure sealants (FS)

This simple restorative procedure has been included in this section on caries control, as it helps to modify local factors that affect the onset and progress of caries and its lesions, namely eradicating caries susceptible, deep fissures/pits on posterior occlusal surfaces of high risk patients. There are two types of FS materials:

● *Resin-based*: visible light-cured systems based on methacrylate resin composite chemistry detailed in Chapter 6. These resins are only lightly filled in order to permit a readily flowable consistency, so creating a void-free infill of deeper fissures. Teeth need to be isolated to obtain moisture control, acid-etched, and the FS is micro-mechanically retained to the enamel surface and light cured (see Chapter 7, Table 7.2).

● *GIC-based:* GICs can be used to bond chemically to the 10% polyacrylic acid-conditioned enamel surface. These materials are more

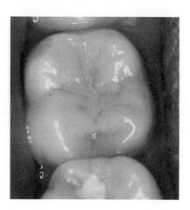

Figure 4.3 A glass ionomer fissure sealant on the occlusal surface of a mandibular molar. (Courtesy of the late Dr J W McLean.)

soluble than the resin-based systems, but do leach fluoride ions which may have a cariostatic effect (see Figure 4.3).

Evidence-based systematic reviews have concluded that there is no clinically significant advantage of one or the other sealant types, although it appears that the resin-based sealants may have increased longevity in clinical use due to easier application and better wear resistance.

The detailed clinical procedure of placing a fissure sealant is described in Chapter 7 (Table 7.2). The indications are as follows:

● In high risk, caries active adolescents, fissure sealing all erupting molars may be advised as a preventive measure.

● In high risk, young adults where there is evidence of caries on molar teeth which need restoration, other susceptible occlusal fissures may be sealed as a precaution.

● In low risk, caries inactive patients with good oral hygiene and minimal/no plaque deposits (checked with disclosing solutions), FS are not generally indicated.

● Young patients with deep fissure patterns, who may otherwise be susceptible due to dietary or other local factors changing (e.g. mentally/physically disabled, patient undergoing extensive orthodontic treatment, medically compromised).

● Cleaned teeth which can be easily isolated using a rubber dam (see Chapters 5 and 7). Saliva contamination during placement may lead to premature complete loss of the sealant restoration or leakage at the margins of a partially debonded restoration, which might then predispose to active caries.

Preventive resin restoration (PRR)/sealant restoration/invasive fissure sealant This is placed after minimally excavating existing occlusal caries, up to the enamel–dentine junction. The PRR restores the cavity with a suitable adhesive restorative material (composite or GIC) followed with an overlying fissure sealant which extends onto the unrestored fissures on the remaining sound portion of the occlusal surface (see Chapter 7, Table 7.3).

4.3 Toothwear control (and lesion prevention)

4.3.1 Process

The control and prevention of toothwear and its lesions is intimately linked with managing the aetiological factors of erosion, attrition, and abrasion discussed in Chapters 1 and 2. The patient's understanding and motivation is vital to the ultimate successful control of toothwear. The aetiological factors must be identified (targeted history and examination) and behaviour subsequently modified (with positive suggestion) in order to remove the causative factor(s). For example, high intake of carbonated drinks/acidic fruit juices over a prolonged period can be adjusted by suggesting that initially, one in three drinks could be tap water and then after 1 month, alternate drinks etc, so gradually reducing the primary causative factor.

4.3.2 Lesions

Once structural tooth surface loss has occurred, it cannot be reversed. Early, asymptomatic lesions in enamel (or just into dentine) may be left untreated. Monitoring and recall of patients with pathological toothwear not requiring immediate operative intervention is discussed in Chapter 8. More extensive tooth loss (accompanied by symptoms including sensitivity, aesthetic considerations and functional difficulties) can be repaired, depending on the severity, with direct, adhesive aesthetic restorations or with indirect, extracoronal restorations (see Figure 4.4). Important factors including the longevity of the protective restorations placed, and changes in the vertical dimension have to be taken into account in the restorative care plan, details of which are beyond the scope of this book.

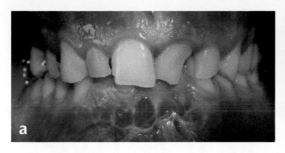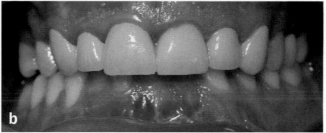

Figure 4.4 (**a**) Preoperative anterior view of a patient with erosion-attrition toothwear caused by gastro-oesophageal reflux disease. (**b**) Anterior view after treatment with metal-ceramic indirect crowns on UR3 to UL3.

Q4.4i: What might the presenting complaints have been?

Q4.4iii: Do you know what might have caused the scar on the anterior mandibular mucosae?

Q4.4ii: The long-term tooth loss has caused a loss in occlusal vertical dimension (see Chapter 5). What clues are present in these images to indicate this process has occurred?

4

4.4 Answers to self-test questions

Q4.1: What might be the possible aetiology of this degree of caries attack?

A: Long-term poor diet and oral hygiene. This appearance is also a presentation of recreational drug-induced caries in young adults – possibly methamphetamine or methadone use (a viscous, sugary syrup).

Q4.2: How can you distinguish these lesions from white spot carious lesions?

A: The site – discrete white spot lesions are usually found closer to the enamel–dentine junction and sites associated with plaque stagnation. These lesions are present across the incisal third of the labial surface and not associated with plaque.

Q4.4i: What might the presenting complaints have been?

A: Poor appearance, sharp edges of the incisors cutting the tongue, teeth fracturing, sensitivity.

Q4.4ii: The long-term tooth loss has caused a loss in occlusal vertical dimension (see Chapter 5). What clues are present in these images to indicate this process has occurred?

A: Note the step up in the line of the attached gingivae of the mandible subjacent to the lower incisors – this is the classic appearance of *dentoalveolar compensation* that has occurred in an attempt to maintain the vertical relationship between the maxillary and mandibular teeth.

Q4.4iii: Do you know what might have caused the scar on the anterior mandibular mucosae?

A: Postoperative scar after fixation of fractured mandible with a bone plate several years ago.

5

The practice of operative dentistry

Chapter contents

5.1 The dental team

All the members of the dental team have a part to play in patient management and comprise the lead dentist (plus other colleagues in the dental practice), the dental nurse, hygienist, receptionist, laboratory technician, and possibly a dental therapist. In the UK, registered dental nurses can take further qualifications in teaching, oral health education, and radiography, and can specialize in other aspects of dentistry including orthodontics, oral surgery, sedation, and special care.

If the dentist wishes to have a second specialist opinion regarding a difficult diagnosis, formulating a care plan or even executing it, they may refer the patient to a specialist dentist working in another practice or to a hospital-based consultant specialist in restorative dentistry. These specialists have undergone further postgraduate clinical and academic training and gained qualifications enabling them to be registered as specialists with the General Dental Council (GDC – UK) in their specific trained fields, e.g. endodontics, periodontics, prosthodontics, or have further specialist training in restorative dentistry. The lead dentist will act as a central hub in the wheel of patient management, possibly outsourcing different aspects of work to relevant specialist colleagues, as spokes of that wheel.

5.2 The dental surgery

This is the operating environment where patients are diagnosed and treated. The operator and nurse work closely together. To be successful, they must build up an understanding of how each other works. The surgery consists of a dental operating chair with an attached or mobile bracket table carrying the rotary instruments and 3-1 air/water syringe (and possibly the light-cure unit and ultrasonic scaler), work surfaces (which should be as clutter-free as possible for good quality infection control – see later), cupboards for storage and two sinks, one for normal handwashing and another for decontaminating soiled instruments prior to sterilization. Often a surgery will also house an X-ray unit for taking intraoral radiographs. Most surgeries are designed to accommodate right-handed practitioners, in terms of the location of many of the instruments and controls. In larger surgeries there may be space to accommodate a table/desk and comfortable chair where the initial verbal consultation may occur before moving to the dental chair for the clinical examination.

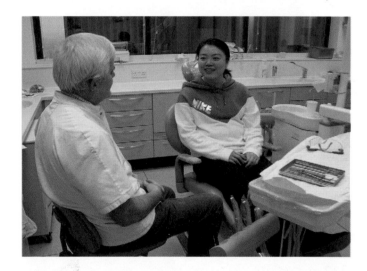

Figure 5.1 Dentist and patient positioning during the consultation. Note how the dentist is sitting slightly in front of the patient and at the same eye level. This positioning enables the patient to feel more comfortable and relaxed.

5.2.1 Positioning the dentist, patient, and nurse

All three must be positioned for maximum comfort, visibility and access whilst maintaining a healthy posture. Initially, the dentist and patient should be sitting at equal eye level, face to face (see Figure 5.1).

The patient is then reclined in the dental chair into a near horizontal position and the height of the chair adjusted so that the patient's head is level with the dentist's mid-sternum, whose knees are placed beneath the patient's headrest. The dentist should sit with their back straight and upper arms vertical with elbows bent at right angles. Thighs should be near-parallel to the floor and knees bent at right angles, with feet firmly placed flat on the floor (see Figure 5.2).

For a right-handed dentist, the nurse should sit to the left of the patient, facing the patient, sitting approximately 10–15 cm higher than the dentist to aid their direct vision into the oral cavity. The nurse's chair may have a foot bar and a swivel back rest that can be moved round to support the nurse when assisting the dentist intraorally. If the patient's head in the dental chair is represented by a clockface with 12 o'clock between the patient's eyes, the dentist can move between 8 o'clock (to view the lower right quadrant with direct vision and the patient slightly more upright in the chair) and 1 o'clock, and the nurse from 1 to 4 o'clock positions (see Figure 5.3). These positions may be reversed for the left-handed operator, assuming that the surgery is designed with this in mind. Some dental chairs are designed so that the nurse's suction and operator's bracket table/mobile cart may be transposed.

5

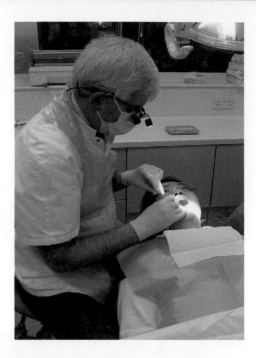

Figure 5.2 Dentist operating position with the patient reclined in the dental chair. Note how the operator's elbows are bent at 90° and the back is straight and shoulders relaxed.

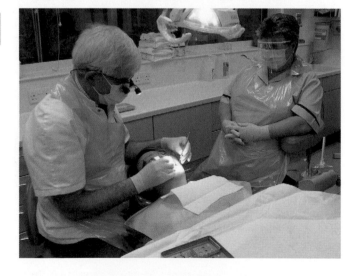

Figure 5.3 The initial positions of the dentist and nurse during the intraoral examination. See text for details.

The patient can facilitate direct intraoral vision by moving their head. The dentist should ask and gently guide the movement, a right head turn to view the upper left buccal quadrant, tipping head down to view the mandibular dentition and lifting the chin up to view the maxillary dentition.

5.2.2 Lighting

Good quality illumination is vital in order to work in a patient's mouth. This is usually afforded by the overhead chair light fitted with daylight-simulating light bulbs. These lights may be focused onto the patient's face and mouth by correct spatial positioning and alignment (some cast a horizontal dark shadow if incorrectly focused). Light handles must be covered with disposable shields for infection control purposes. LED headlights can be worn by the operator, focusing a beam of shadowless light in the direction of the dentist's gaze (see Figure 5.4). Care needs to be taken when working with resin composites as these can be prematurely light cured by intense LED outputs (with narrow emission spectra around 470 nm). An orange filter can be used to prevent this.

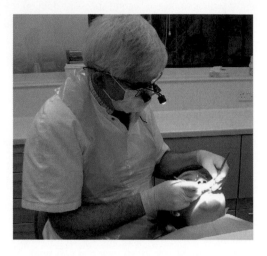

Figure 5.4 The dentist is using an LED headlight to help illuminate his field of view, without shadows.

5.2.3 Zoning

For infection control purposes, the dental surgery must be divided into zones for clinical notes/clean instruments and dirty instruments. It is important that these zones are designed with practicality in mind as thoroughfare between and through them should be kept to a minimum to prevent cross-contamination between zones. An example in a hospital setting is shown in Figure 5.5, but variations will obviously be found in different dental practice surgeries. Dirty zones (areas that are likely to become contaminated by direct contact, aerosols, or splatter during treatment procedures) include:

- Bracket table and handle
- Dental handpiece unit, connectors, and switches
- Dental chair head rest
- Light handles/switch
- Chair handle controls
- Suction connectors
- Spittoon.

These zones must be cleaned and disinfected appropriately between patients. To aid this process, most of the above can be covered with clear plastic wrap (cling film) or plastic sleeves, which are removed, zones cleaned and plastic wrap replaced between patients.

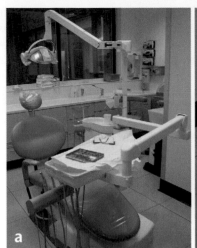
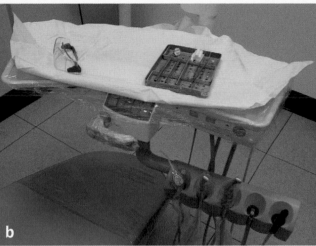
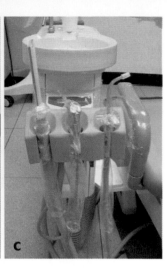

Figure 5.5 The infection control barriers placed when setting up a dental surgery. (**a**) An overview of the surgery, (**b**) the bracket table, and (**c**) the spittoon area. Note the use of disposable suction tips and barrier protection on all tubing.

5.3 Infection control/personal protective equipment (PPE)

Current guidelines require the dentist and nurse to be dressed in short sleeve tunic/uniforms, no neckties that hang loosely from the neck and no jewellery (except wedding bands). Footwear should cover the tops of feet. Standard infection control practice against blood-borne, air-borne, and other body fluid-borne pathogens is outlined in Table 5.1. With regard to protecting the patient, a disposable neck towel should be placed over the patient and suitable eye protection must be worn by the patient while in the reclined position (see Figure 5.6).

5

Table 5.1 Infection control procedures for the dental team

Infection control precautions	Comments
Hand hygiene	Soap/detergent and running water; alcohol hand gels before donning and after removing gloves.
Skin dressings	Cuts, abrasions, and skin conditions protected with waterproof dressings.
Sharps handling	Used needles and sharps should be disposed by the user into rigid sharps containers. Only re-sheath needles if using a re-sheathing device/single-handed technique.
Personal protective equipment (PPE)	Reusable protective eyewear worn (goggles with side protection or visors over spectacles) if risk of blood/body fluid splashing to the face. Single-use surgical face masks provide a physical barrier to splashes to the mouth/face. They do not protect the wearer from aerosol inhalation. Respirator-type masks can be used to protect against aerosol inhalation. Single-use gloves: natural rubber latex (NRL, non-powdered), nitrile (acrylonitrile)/polychloroprene (Tactylon) gloves should be worn (non-allergenic). NRL can result in development of latex hypersensitivity – delayed type IV (contact dermatitis, rhinitis, conjunctivitis up to 48 hours after exposure) or, less commonly, immediate type I (asthma, urticaria, laryngeal oedema, anaphylactic shock usually within 30 minutes after exposure). Single-use plastic aprons to prevent contamination of clothing.
Blood/body fluid spillages	Dealt with using hypochlorite granules and appropriate PPE.
Clinical waste handling	Infectious, hazardous waste disposed of in yellow clinical waste bags.
Instruments	Single-use sharp instruments disposed of in appropriate sharps container. Reusable instruments must undergo decontamination prior to sterilization (see below).

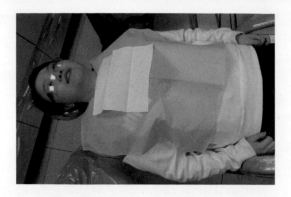

Figure 5.6 Patient in a reclined position wearing eye protection and a disposable bib and neck towel.

5.3.1 Decontamination and sterilization procedures

The days of locating the sterilizing unit in the corner of the surgery are numbered. Separate sterilization facilities for reusable equipment are required (either in a decontamination unit or a segregated area within the surgery) with contaminated entry and clean exit pathways clearly demarcated. This area should be separated into dirty, sterilization, and clean zones. Instruments need to be washed manually and placed in an ultrasonic bath to remove debris. A thermal washer-disinfector is recommended. Dental handpieces require lubrication before and after sterilization, using manual aerosols or by an air-driven cleaning/lubricating unit (see Figure 5.7).

Once this decontamination cycle is completed, non-vacuum (downward/gravity displacement bench-top steam) or vacuum bench-top steam sterilization (recommended for wrapped/unwrapped, hollow lumen items) is required before individual instruments are dried (so preventing long-term corrosion of carbon steel instruments) and finally bagged in sterile packets and stored in the clean zone. Conventional default settings for most steam sterilizers are 134–137 °C held for 3 minutes at a pressure of 2.5 bar. In hospitals, central sterilizing facilities take on this role and soiled instruments are carefully packaged.

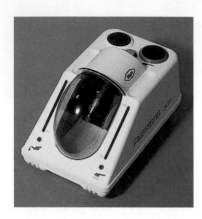

Figure 5.7 An automatic handpiece cleaning unit which is connected to the air supply. The shield at the front is rotated out of the way and the handpiece plugged onto the connector. A detergent is then flushed through the handpiece followed by oil, both of which come from refillable containers at the back of the unit. This is a more efficient and quicker system than using aerosols.

5.4 Patient safety and risk management

During operative dental procedures patient safety is of paramount importance. Accidents will happen, but the risk of these occurring must be minimized or even eradicated at all costs – this is known as *risk management*. In terms of sustaining injury/harm during a dental procedure, the vulnerable areas of the patient include their eyes, airway, and soft tissues. The damage can be caused by inappropriate

Table 5.2 A summary of the potential sites/type of patient injury, causes, and methods used by the dental team to prevent them occurring

Patient	Aetiology of injury	Type of injury	Prevention
Eyes	Sharp instruments slipping/burs fracturing, fragments of restoration, aerosolized dental materials/body fluids.	Laceration, burn, infection.	Protective glasses (with side covers) worn when patient supine.
Airway	Small instruments (fractured burs, RCT files), indirect restorations (crowns, inlays), implant components, extracted teeth/fragments.	Inhalation or swallowed. Lung infection, blockage of URT airway.	Rubber dam; safety chains/floss tied to small instruments; gauze squares placed intraorally to cover back of throat.
Soft tissues (lips, mucosae, tongue)	Caustic dental materials (acid etch, hypochlorite), sharp instruments (including needles), rotary burs, heat, aggressive retraction of soft tissues, compressed air introduced into open wounds; anaesthetized tissues.	Burns, lacerations, grazes, surgical emphysema.	Rubber dam placed correctly with sufficient seal; proper use/maintenance of handpieces/burs; single-use needles – *do not bend*. Avoid directing air jets into broken mucosae, exposed root canals.

RCT, root canal therapy; URT, upper respiratory tract.

use/maintenance of sharp instruments, burs, small instruments, and improper use/handling of dental materials. Table 5.2 outlines the sites, aetiology, and types of injury that might be sustained and methods to prevent them occurring.

5.4.1 Management of minor injuries

In all cases of injury, the patient must be informed and the events documented comprehensively in the patient's notes.

- *Eyes*: if debris enters the eyes (patient or member of the dental team), immediate washing in an eye-bath with sterile water is essential with follow-up medical care if required.

- *Airway*: if an inhalational blockage occurs, stand the patient bent at the hips and firmly slap the patient's back to help dislodge the object from the oropharynx. Check the object has not been sucked up the high volume aspirator (if in use). If the object cannot be accounted for, and the patient is not sure whether they have swallowed it, a chest radiograph will be required to help localize the foreign object in either the bronchi, lungs, oesophagus, or the stomach (see Figure 5.8). Follow-up medical attention will be required, especially for the former, as a bronchoscopy may be indicated.

- *Soft tissues*: Haemostasis of cuts and abrasions must be obtained. Cuts to the lips or mucosae may need sutures. Caustic sodium hypochlorite burns (caused by a leaking rubber dam in root canal therapy (RCT)) may require medical attention and a suitable dressing to promote healing without scarring. Patients with inferior alveolar nerve anaesthesia should be warned of the persistent numbness for several hours after treatment and to take care in avoiding biting/chewing their lower lip or having hot food or drink in case of burning themselves.

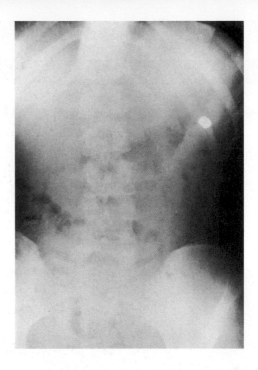

Figure 5.8 Radiograph showing a gold crown in a patient's stomach (courtesy of Professor A H R Rowe).

Q5.8: Can you spot the gold crown?

5

5.5 Dental aesthetics and shade selection

The advent in the early 1960s and continued development of adhesive, tooth-coloured restorative materials have raised patients' expectations with regard to high quality aesthetic results when it comes to restoring teeth to form and function, especially in the anterior 'aesthetic zone' (UR4 – UL4). An aesthetically pleasing dental result depends on numerous complex and interlinked factors including:

- The three-dimensional shape of the tooth
- The inherent shade of the tooth
- The surface form and finish of the tooth
- The morphology of the surrounding periodontal tissues
- The occlusal plane and relationship with adjacent/opposing teeth.

The dental materials that can offer shades and characteristics that closely match natural tooth in descending order are:

- Dental porcelains (indirect – made by a dental technician in a laboratory from casts poured from dental impressions and finally cemented in/on the tooth)
- Dental composites (direct – placed at chairside, and indirect (made in the laboratory))
- Glass ionomer cements (direct – include resin-modified and polyacid-modified composites).

5.5.1 Colour perception

The human brain is able to perceive intrinsic physical properties of incident light sensed by the eye. In order to communicate these, colour scales have been devised. One of the earliest was the system from A H Munsell, which comprised three elements: the dominant wavelength (*hue*), the excitation purity (*chroma*), and its luminous reflectance (*value*) (Table 5.3).

Table 5.3 The intrinsic physical properties of light perceivable by the human eye according to the Munsell colour space classification

Property of light	Comments
Hue (wavelength)	Wavelength of coloured light translated as its actual colour, e.g. red, green, blue, etc. Figure 5.9 shows the Vitapan Classical shade guide tabs arranged in the four-lettered groups according to hue. A: more reddish-brown, B: yellow; C: yellow-grey; and D: more reddish-grey.
Chroma (saturation)	Strength/dominance of the colour (hue). Light or dark shade. Figure 5.9 shows the Classical shade tabs arranged with increasing chroma (1–4) in each of the hue (colour) groups (A–D).
Value (greyness)	Luminosity of the colour (the level of black or white – its *greyness*). Figures 5.10 and 5.11 show the shade tabs arranged in descending order of value. Enamel thickness is the major contributor to the value of a tooth.

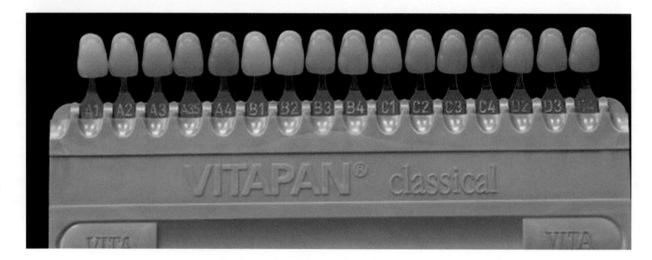

Figure 5.9 The Vitapan Classical shade guide tabs, arranged in four groups A–D according to hue (colour) and within each hue, a range of increasing chroma, 1–4.

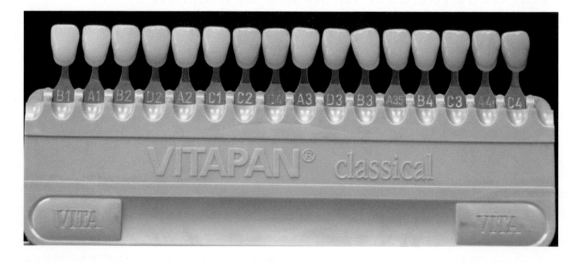

Figure 5.10 The Vitapan Classical shade guide tabs arranged in order of value (high (whiter) to low (darker)).

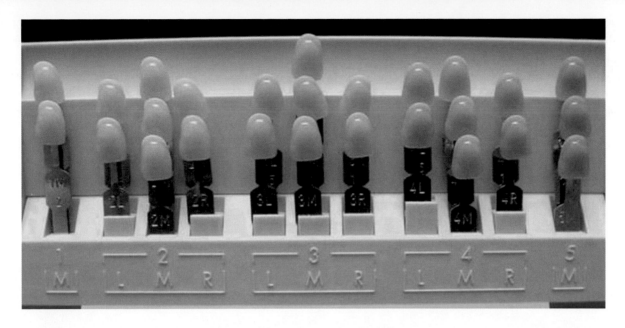

Figure 5.11 The Vitapan 3D-Master shade guide with value graded from 1 to 5 (light to dark), three chroma choices within the value groups 2, 3, and 4 and the individual hue (yellow-red).

However, the human tooth is heterogeneous and the pulp, dentine, enamel, their interfaces, and relative thicknesses along with their changing histological structure all play a part in overall perception of the shade by affecting the interaction between the light and the tooth structure. When attempting to mimic the shade of a tooth, the inherent structure of the restorative material and how it affects the physical characteristics of incident light must be considered, i.e. the reflectance, translucency, opacity, and fluorescence. As the Munsell classification does not take these factors into account, another classification was devised by the Commission Internationale de l'Eclairage (CIE): the CIE L* a* b* colour space. This classification applies the amount of red, green, and blue colours used; L* measures lightness (0–100, black-white) and CIE a* and b*, the relative hue and chroma (a*, levels of red(+)-green(–); b*, levels of yellow(+)-blue(–)). This system permits numerical quantification and calculation of colour, expressed in units that can be related to visual perception and clinical significance. This scale is used in research studies into colour and also the electronic shade guides (see later). The properties of the restorative material that can help mimic these interactions include:

- *Refractive index*: refraction is the change in direction of light due to it entering a medium of different density. Different materials have different refractive indices. The difference between the refractive indices of two materials determines how opaque or translucent one appears when observed from the other. The opacity of a composite depends on the difference between the refractive index of the composite material and the refractive index of air.

- *Scattering coefficient*: scattering is the loss of light due to the reversal of its direction. The scattering coefficient varies with wavelength of the light and the nature of the colorant layer of a composite. A composite with a greater refractive index (dependent on the polymer matrix, size/type/amount of filler particles, aluminium/zirconium/titanium oxide opacifiers present) will appear more opaque.

- *Absorption coefficient*: absorption is the taking up of light by a material. The absorption coefficient also depends on the wavelength of light and the nature of the colorant layer of the composite. The greater the absorption coefficient, the more opaque and intensely coloured the composite will appear.

When restoring a tooth with a direct composite it is advisable to use layering techniques in order to copy these variations that occur within the tooth. In a young tooth, the thicker enamel will affect the value and hue, with the dentine contributing towards the chromatic aspect of its shade. As the tooth ages and the enamel thins, so the dentine and pulp have more of an influence on the hue, with enamel contributing primarily to the value of the final shade. The enamel–dentine junction (EDJ) contributes to the fluorescent characteristics (which can be added in a layering technique using coloured tints and stains). The quality of the surface finish and form will affect the reflectivity of incident light; using a more flowable, translucent low filler particle content composite will assist in producing a smooth, blemish-free surface after careful polishing (see later). Some manufacturers provide their own shade guide with their layering composite system to simplify the choice of dentine and enamel shades, often calibrated to the Vitapan Classical system.

5.5.2 Clinical tips for shade selection

- Avoid brightly coloured neck towels. It is helpful to use a light blue neck cloth. Select shade before placing rubber dam as teeth become lighter as they dry out.

- Ask patients to remove bright lipstick or other obstacles, such as hoods or hats, which may affect incident light/shadows.

5

- Schedule aesthetic restoration appointments early in the morning if possible to avoid eye fatigue.

- The light source should be diffuse, not direct. Natural daylight where possible. Try to avoid conventional fluorescent light sources.

- Fan the shade guide past the patient's mouth and pick the closest tab. Do not stare. Rest your eyes occasionally. After selecting the hue, squinting/half-closing your eyes will aid the determination of the value.

- Cold sterilize shade guides to prevent damaging them.

- Shade taking should be carried out after prophylaxis but before tooth isolation and preparation, since dehydration can artificially lighten the natural tooth shade.

- Select the body shade by examining the centre portion of the tooth (see Figure 5.12). Check with mouth open and closed (lips parted) for anterior dentition.

- Choose the composite shade most closely approximating the centre portion of the shade guide (see Figure 5.12). Custom-made resin composite shade tabs can be constructed from the specific brand of material used by the dentist. Using glass slabs, various thicknesses of each shade of resin composite can be cured and labelled and then used subsequently for shade selection.

- Place and cure the chosen shade of composite on the tooth surface to be restored, using the correct thickness of material (see Figure 5.12). No etch or bond required. Patient can use a face mirror to help check the shade of material selected.

5

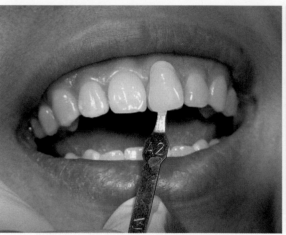 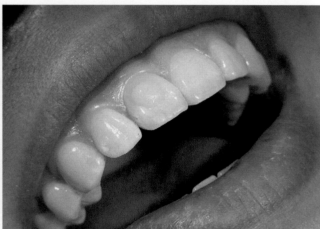

Figure 5.12 Shade assessment of UR1 using a shade tab (left image) assessing the shade from the body of the tab and tooth and then placing the resin composite on the unetched labial surface of the tooth to make the final assessment, ensuring the tooth is not dehydrated.

As well as the visual shade guides depicted in Figures 5.9–5.11, there are electronic shade detectors which shine an incident beam of light onto the relevant tooth and then numerically analyse the reflected light. Care has to be taken when assessing particularly translucent incisal edges as these instruments can mis-report the translucency as a greyer overall shade as a significant proportion of the light passes through the tooth rather than being reflected back.

5.6 Moisture control

This is the ability to regulate the fluid environment within the oral cavity and around the individual teeth being operated on. Fluids include water, saliva, gingival exudate, and blood.

5.6.1 Why?

Moisture control is required:

- To permit proper placement of all restorations – excessive fluids have a detrimental effect on the adhesion and/or physical properties of all direct plastic restorations, but especially those relying on adhesive bonding.

- To prevent contamination of the restorative procedure – caries removal, direct pulp capping, RCT, and adhesive bonding.

- To improve patient comfort – removing accumulated fluids produced by dental handpieces, 3-1 syringes, and salivary flow.

5.6.2 Techniques

- *Aspiration*: fluids can be evacuated using a single-use saliva ejector by the nurse, the dentist or even the patient (see Figure 5.13). Plastic tips can be bent into a curved shape to adapt the contours of the lips

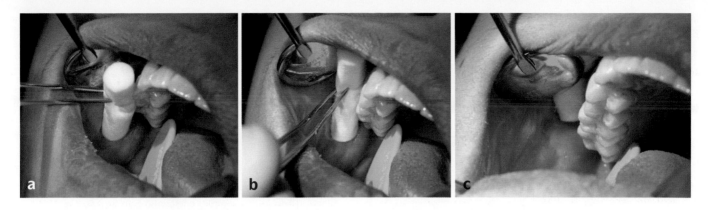

Figure 5.13 (a–c) Series of images showing how to place successfully a cotton wool roll into the maxillary right buccal sulcus – note the way it is rotated into position so ensuring it will stay in place. A blue flanged disposable saliva ejector tip has been placed lingually to help retract the tongue.

and oral cavity so accessing the buccal or lingual sulci while simultaneously retracting these tissues.

- *Cotton wool rolls (cellulose pads)*: used to absorb fluids and retract lips or cheeks. Placed over salivary duct orifices, upper buccal sulci (parotid ducts), lingual sulci (submandibular and sublingual ducts; see Figures 5.13, 5.14).

- *Rubber dam*: a thin latex (or equivalent) perforated sheet that isolates single or groups of teeth so allowing the best control of moisture. Its advantages/disadvantages are listed in Table 5.4, and the equipment required to place rubber dam isolation is described in Figures 5.15–5.18

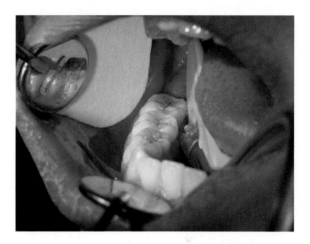

Figure 5.14 A cellulose pad has been used to absorb moisture from the right parotid duct within the maxillary right buccal sulcus.

Table 5.4 The advantages and disadvantages of placing and using rubber dam for moisture control

Advantages	Disadvantages
Controlled isolation of the teeth from fluids (reducing adverse effects on bonding/physical properties).	More difficult to communicate with the patient.
Reduced bacterial contamination (caries removal, pulp capping, root canal therapy (RCT)).	Some patients dislike the feeling of claustrophobia (may be reduced by relieving the dam away from the nasal passages).
Patient airway protection from inhalation/swallowing instruments (restorations, burs, endodontic files, wedges); orofacial soft tissue protection from chemical agents (acid-etch gel, dilute hypochlorite solution used in RCT).	Attaching the rubber dam to teeth with clamps can cause pain and some postoperative pain for several hours.
Can act as barrier protection from fluid-borne pathogen transfer from patient to dentist.	Poorly fitted clamps can cause damage to ceramic crowns (chipping).
Positive psychological experience/improved comfort for some patients. A feeling of detachment/separation from the operation.	Care needed to check medical history for latex allergies for both patient and dentist. Non-latex containing dams are available.
Can aid in tissue retraction and so improve direct vision – keeps oral mucosae and tongue separate from the operation field.	In inexperienced hands, rubber dam placement can be difficult and time-consuming. Once mastered this problem is alleviated, however.
Once in place, rubber dam can speed up the procedure for the dental team.	

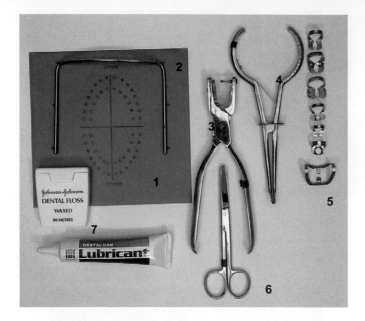

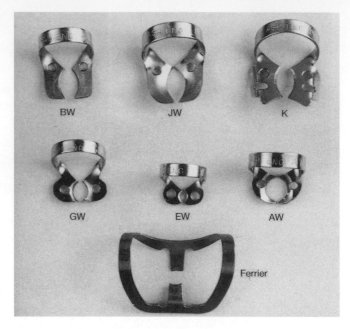

Figure 5.15 Rubber dam equipment comprising:

1. A 15 cm square dark green rubber sheet (with the position for the perforation holes stamped on using an ink-stamp). The rubber resists tearing and grips the tooth surface. Dark colours are used to contrast with the teeth and torn fragments, often interproximally, can be detected and removed.

2. Metal rubber dam frame holds the free edges away from the face/mouth. The dam is stretched around the tines on the frame itself, keeping it under tension.

3. Rubber dam hole punch – creates a clean cut perforation of three diameters (corresponding to incisors, premolars, and molars)

4. Rubber dam clamp forceps – used to place, adjust, and remove clamps from teeth.

5. Rubber dam clamps – metal clips that grasp the coronal neck of the tooth holding the dam down. Can be winged or wingless (see Figure 5.16).

6. Scissors to cut excess dam away from the nose and when removing the dam, interproximally.

7. Waxed dental floss and a water-based dam lubricant – both aid the transition of the dam through tight contact points. Floss can act as a ligature, tying the dam down at the gingival margin.

Figure 5.16 A close-up view of metal rubber dam clamps, comprising two jaws joined by a curved connecting arm. The two holes accommodate the clamp forceps, which allow the opposing jaws to be separated when placing/removing them over the crown bulbosity. BW, JW, K, and AW clamps are molar patterned (AW is more retentive for partially erupted crowns), GW is used for canines/premolars and EW is configured for any other smaller tooth. The K clamp is winged – it has two extensions onto which the dam can be placed prior to inserting the dam and clamp together onto the tooth (useful when isolating just one tooth in the arch). The remaining wingless clamps must be first placed onto the teeth followed by the manual application of the dam over them. The Ferrier clamp is used for retracting gingivae when isolating anterior teeth, working in the cervical area (care is needed not to traumatize the gingivae and cause blood contamination of the field, see Chapter 7).

5.6.3 Rubber dam placement – the practical steps

Figures 5.17 and 5.18 show how a rubber dam can be placed on and then removed from an upper molar using either a wingless (see Figure 5.17) or winged clamp (see Figure 5.18). Some patients may need local anaesthesia/topical anaesthesia to dull the pain of the clamp on the tooth/periodontium. If a matrix band is required to help contour the final restoration, the rubber dam clamp may need to be removed as it will get in the way of the circumferential or sectional matrix system (see later). In this situation, the matrix band will take over the role of the clamp in holding the dam in position while the material is packed into place.

For anterior teeth, there is less need to use clamps as the tight contact points can be sufficient to retain the well-adapted dam interdentally or else a thin strip of rubber dam cut from the peripheral excess, alternatively proprietary rubber wedgets can be used by 'flossing' them beyond the contact points. Floss ligatures may also be used. If the contact points are too tight initially for even floss to pass, then interdental pre-wedging with a wooden wedge for 5 minutes before placing the dam will usually cause enough tooth movement within its periodontal ligament (and that of the adjacent tooth) to allow the dam to pass between. Careful use of the anterior Ferrier clamp is required so as not to traumatize the gingival margins.

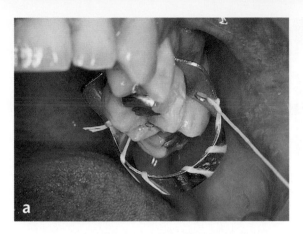

Figure 5.17 (**a**) A wingless JW clamp placed on the UL6. Clamp forceps were used to open the jaws of the clamp sufficiently to allow it to pass over the bulbosity of the crown. Note the floss tied through both clamp holes and coiled around the connector arm. This makes any clamp fragments retrievable if the connector arm fractures under tension, in use. The connector arm is placed distally to prevent the clamp from blocking access to the tooth.

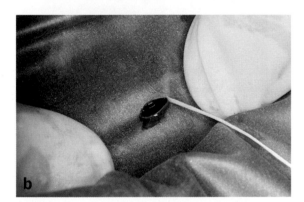

Figure 5.17 (**b**) The dam is gently stretched by the dentist to widen the lubricated perforation and the free end of the floss is passed through the hole.

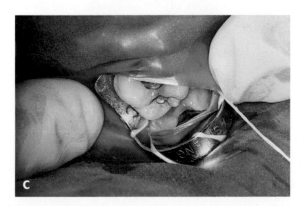

Figure 5.17 (**c**) The dam is stretched over the connector arm first and then over the two clamps embracing the tooth. The nurse can help by keeping the floss taught throughout the procedure.

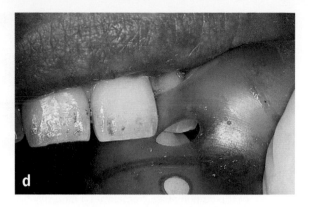

Figure 5.17 (**d**) The dam is then 'knifed' though the contact areas of the remaining teeth to be isolated in the UL quadrant.

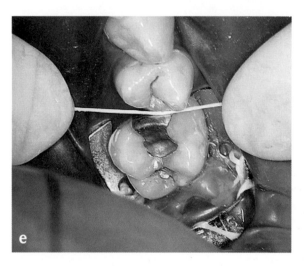

Figure 5.17 (**e**) Floss is used to work the dam down through the mesial contact area of the UL6.

5

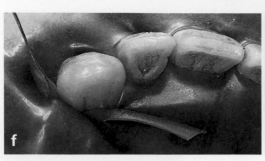

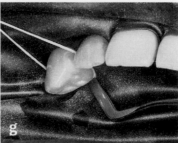

Figure 5.17 (**f**) A strip of dam has been wedged in the distal contact of the UR3 to hold the anterior portion of the dam in place. Sometimes a naturally tight contact may suffice. The dam is yet to be inverted around the cervical margins of the teeth. (**g**) Alternatively, a floss ligature could be used to the same effect, using a flat plastic instrument to ensure palatal placement apical to the maximum bulbosity of the crown and inverting the dam simultaneously. It will not always be clinically necessary to isolate so many teeth if only working on the UL quadrant.

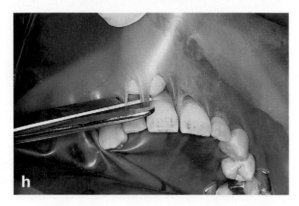

Figure 5.17 (**h**) When removing the dam, it is pulled buccally and cut interdentally using scissors. Note the operator's finger beneath the dam protecting the patient's lip. The frame, dam, and clamp are removed together and checked for completeness.

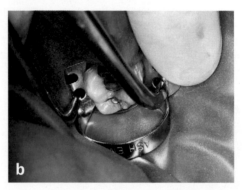

Figure 5.18 (**b**) Clamp and rubber dam being secured to the UL6 as one, using the clamp forceps (note the two pairs of holes to engage the forceps). The nurse can assist the process by gently retracting the loose rubber dam edges to aid vision. Again, the connector arm is placed distal to the tooth being operated upon so as not to block access to instrumentation/visibility.

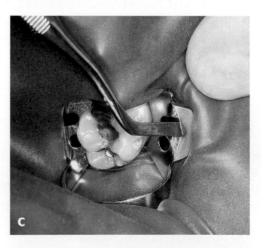

Figure 5.18 (**c**) The dam is disengaged from the wings using a flat plastic instrument and the contact areas will be flossed to ensure interdental adaptation of the dam.

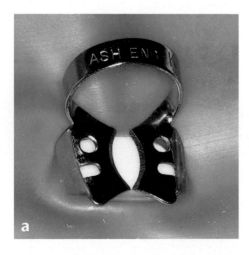

Figure 5.18 (**a**) K clamp (winged molar) with the wings engaged in the lubricated perforation in the dam, outside the mouth.

Q5.18: Can you spot a clinical omission in Figure 5.18?

5.7 Magnification

Visual magnification aiding clinical examination/operating can be achieved using *magnifiers* or *dental loupes*. A selection can be seen in Figure 5.19. In terms of optical physics, there are two aspects to consider with regard to their clinical application: the *depth of field* (or *focus*) and *field of view* (or *field width*).

- *Depth of field (DoF)*: equates to the distance the operator can move towards or away from the object tooth while keeping the image in clear focus. If this range is limited, procedures become tiring as the operator and patient must always remain at a fixed distance from each other with minimal leeway of movement of either person before the view becomes blurred. For a given magnification, the DoF depends on the f-number of the lens (aperture diameter); ↑ f-number (↓ aperture) leads to an ↑ DoF.

- *Field of view (FoV)*: the angular extent of the observable image viewed through the fixed-magnification loupes. Normal unaided human binocular vision (with depth perception) permits 140° FoV. With increasing magnification, this is greatly reduced, e.g. 3× magnification with loupes may only permit a clear, sharp view of the object tooth and one either side (depending on the actual optics of the loupes). This can make introducing dental instruments into the operating field difficult and will require the dentist to look away from the loupes' view to do this.

For general dentistry, 2–3× magnification is usually satisfactory but for endodontics, 4–5× magnification can be used to help detect root canal orifices and fine root canals. Good visual discrimination in dental procedures requires good depth perception, which in turn requires

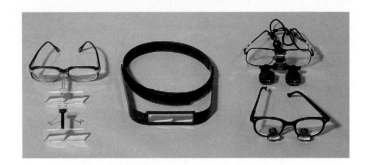

Figure 5.19 A selection of magnification loupes. The first three are the cheapest and have the simplest optics, clipping onto existing spectacles/safety glasses or being secured with a head loop. The two on the right are more expensive. The top right pair have interchangeable lens blocks and due to their weight, require a head cord for retention. Those on the bottom right have the dentist's fixed interpupillary distance built in as the lenses are cemented through the prescription/safety spectacle lenses. As the magnification optics are closer to the eye, this results in a greater field width and depth of field but at increased expense.

binocular function. To get the most out of the increased magnification, good quality illumination is also vital. Modern magnification systems often can be fitted with halogen or LED lights that are integrated on the frame above the lenses and can be focused on the same focal plane as the lenses (see Figure 5.4). Orange light filters should be used to prevent premature light curing of resin-based materials.

5.8 Instruments used in operative dentistry

Instruments are used to examine, clean, cut, and help restore teeth. The main types of cutting instruments are either hand-held or rotary instruments driven in a handpiece. Other equipment includes fibre-optic lights for illumination, light-curing systems used for polymerization of resin-based materials, new instruments for tooth-cutting/caries removal, and ultrasonic scalers (Table 5.5). These instruments may be reused after suitable decontamination and sterilization procedures, or else are disposable, single-use items.

Table 5.5 Tooth-cutting/caries removal technologies, the substrates acted on and their mechanism of action

Mechanism	Substrate affected	Tooth-cutting technology
Mechanical, rotary	Sound or carious enamel and dentine	SS, CS, diamond, TC and non-metallic burs*
Mechanical, non-rotary	Sound or carious enamel and dentine	Hand instruments (excavators, chisels), air-abrasion, air-polishing†, ultrasonics, sono-abrasion
Chemo-mechanical	Carious dentine	Caridex, Carisolv gel (amino acid-based), Papacarie gel (papain-based), pepsin-based solutions/gels
Photo-ablation	Sound or carious enamel and dentine	Lasers
Others	Bacteria	Photoactive disinfection (PAD), ozone

*Works only on carious dentine; †primarily used for stain-removal.
SS, stainless steel; CS, carbon steel; TC, tungsten carbide.

5.8.1 Hand instruments

Manufactured from medical grade stainless or carbon steel (sometimes with tungsten carbide brazed to the cutting edges for increased longevity of sharpness), the majority of hand instruments are designed with a handle, shank, and blade configuration (see Figure 5.20).

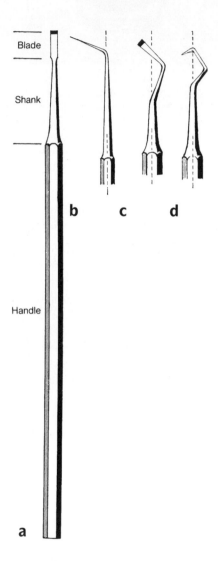

Figure 5.20 **(a)** The parts of a hand instrument. **(b)** A straight probe with a single bend taking the working tip well away from the handle's long axis, so aiding direct vision. **(c)** Two bends in a hatchet. **(d)** Three bends in a Briault probe. Medical grade stainless steel cutting edges can be re-sharpened using a sharpening stone with oil lubricant (fine edge) or a dry abrasive disc (coarse edge). Tungsten carbide tips should be sent to the manufacturer for resharpening.

Hand instruments can be used for the following purposes:

- Oral examination (mouth mirror, selection of dental probes, pair of tweezers):
  - *Mouth mirrors*: front or rear-surfaced (see Figure 5.21)

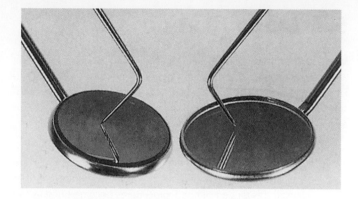

Figure 5.21 Front- and rear-surface mouth mirrors. The left mirror (front-surface) gives a clearer image than the rear-surface 'double' image (right), but is more prone to scratch damage during use and sterilization procedures.

  - *Dental probes*: sharp probes (straight and Briault) are only used for checking restoration margins and carious dentine to be excavated. Round-ended/blunt periodontal probes are used for periodontal examination and assessing the roughness of enamel/occlusal surfaces (see Figure 5.22)

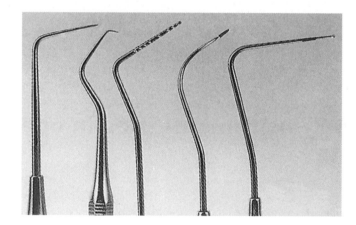

Figure 5.22 A selection of dental probes (from left to right): straight, Briault, Williams', Naber's and CPITN probes.

Q5.22: In which clinical situations might you use each of the probes above?

  - Locking tweezers: to place cotton wool rolls, remove large pieces of intraoral debris.
- With the advent of modern infection control guidelines, disposable examination instruments are now manufactured from plastic to allow single use only (see Figure 5.23).

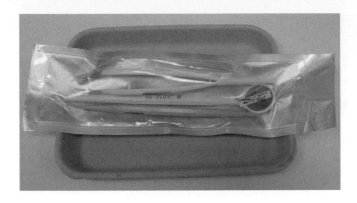

Figure 5.23 Disposable, single-use plastic examination instruments – mirror, probe, and tweezers – in their sterile packaging.

- Periodontal scaling: a selection of *hand-held scalers* (see Figure 5.24) to remove supra- and sub-gingival calculus deposits.

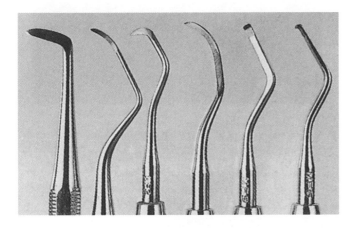

Figure 5.24 A selection of hand-held periodontal scalers (blade and shank visible). Note the angulation of the heads and the extent that the cutting blades are offset from the long axis of the handle.

- Caries removal (excavators, chisels/hatchets/hoes):
  - *Excavators*: instruments with a discoid/ovoid blade sharpened to a cutting edge are used to remove caries and soft temporary restorations. Can also be used to shape plastic restorative materials (see Figure 5.25)
  - *Chisels, hatchets and hoes*: used to remove unsupported enamel/ bevel cavity margins (especially where access for rotary instruments is limited). Hatchets and hoes are similar to chisels in having a straight bevelled cutting edge and are always angled or contra-angled. They differ from one another in that the cutting edge of the hatchet is in the plane of the shank (like an axe), whereas the cutting edge of the hoe lies in an axis at right angles to this plane (as in a gardener's hoe; see Figure 5.26).
- Handling restorative materials (flat plastics, condensers (pluggers), carvers):
  - *Flat plastic instruments*: used for conveying, placing and shaping plastic materials not requiring heavy pressure. Usually made of

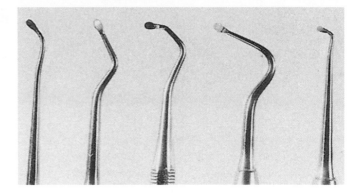

Figure 5.25 A selection of hand excavators (blade and shank visible) – note the different ovoid blade sizes and offset angulations.

Q5.25: What are the advantages of having angulations between the working heads and shanks of these instruments?

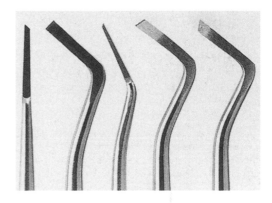

Figure 5.26 A selection of straight and angled chisels (from left to right): straight, hatchet, hoe, and a pair of double-ended gingival margin trimmers.

stainless steel but for composite placement, Teflon-coated or titanium nitride-coated blades confer a useful non-stick property (see Figure 5.27)
  - *Condensers (pluggers)*: smooth surface instruments for packing plastic restorative materials into cavities under pressure (eliminating voids) (see Figure 5.27)
  - *Carving instruments*: sharp/semi-sharp blades carve the shape/contour of the final restoration by cutting/scraping action. Different patterns exist, e.g. Ward's, Half-Hollenback (see Figure 5.27).

5.8.2 Rotary instruments

Dental burs, stones, and cutting and polishing discs are small instruments ('drill bits') gripped firmly by a chuck in a handpiece ('dental drill') powered directly by compressed air, the *air turbine*, or by a separate motor either air or electrically driven, the *low-speed* handpieces.

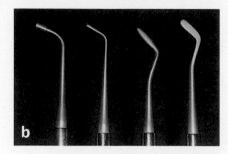

Figure 5.27 (a) Stainless steel and **(b)** titanium nitride-coated (non-stick, gold-coloured) instruments for conveying, placing, and shaping composite materials. Left to right in both images: Guy's pattern condenser (plugger), burnisher (to adapt material to cavity margins), carving instrument (Half-Hollenback pattern), flat plastic.

- *Air turbine ('high-speed') handpieces*: clockwise rotary speeds between 250 000 and 500 000 revolutions per minute (rpm) but relatively low torque, achieved by a small air-driven turbine or rotor mounted in bearings in the head of a contra-angled handpiece. Burs are held via a friction-grip shank, the tip shrouded in water spray and illuminated with an optional fibreoptic light (Figure 5.28).

- *Low-speed handpieces*: two-piece system comprising an electric or air-driven motor coupled to a contra-angled or straight handpiece (rotating clockwise or anticlockwise), with water spray and fibreoptic light; lower speed but higher torque than the air turbine handpiece (see Figure 5.29).

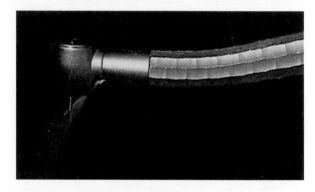

Figure 5.28 Air turbine handpiece in operation showing the directed water spray over the tip of the bur and the fibreoptic light.

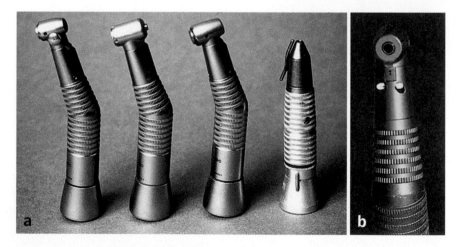

Figure 5.29 (a, b) A selection of low-speed handpieces. From the left:
1:1 contra-angled handpiece used for most procedures. Latch-grip burs are used. Commonly identified with a blue-coloured band on the shank of the handpiece and a blue dot on the head. Speed in the range 400–40 000 rpm.
1:4 speed-increasing handpiece. Friction-grip burs. Operates at 16 000–160 000 rpm. Commonly identified with a red band. Useful for finishing cavity preparations and also finishing restorations.
7:1 speed-reducing handpiece. Latch-grip burs. Used for drilling pin holes and other procedures where slow speed is indicated. Operates at 550–5500 rpm and is commonly identified with a green band.
Straight handpiece that takes straight burs (may be modified to take latch-grip burs). A 1:1 handpiece is identified with a blue band; speed-reducing is identified with a green band. Used to trim temporary restorations and other similar procedures. Usually used outside the mouth.
A fibreoptic light system built into the head of a contra-angled low-speed handpiece.

● *Dental burs* (see Figures 5.30, 5.34), *stones* (see Figure 5.31), and *finishing burs/discs* (see Figures 5.32, 5.33): gripped in handpieces by a quick-release clamping chuck (friction-grip diamond grit/tungsten carbide (TC) cutting blades for air turbine handpieces; latch-grip carbon steel/diamond grit/TC/plastic cutting blades for low-speed handpieces).

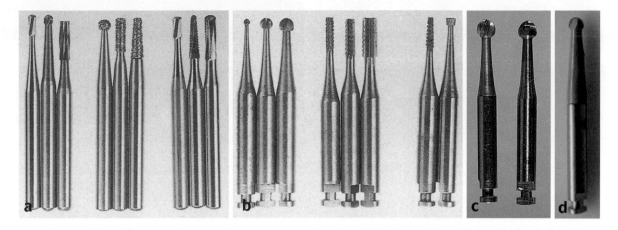

Figure 5.30 A series of eight sets of burs (first three sets, friction-grip for the air turbine, next five sets, latch-grip for the low-speed handpiece). **(a)** Friction-grip: tungsten carbide (TC) ×3, diamond grit (round, straight, tapered) and metal-cutting (serrated cross-cut TC blade) burs. TC and diamond used for cutting sound enamel and dentine, removing existing restorations. Diamond burs can be used to cut ceramic. **(b, c)** Latch-grip, carbon steel: three sizes round (rose-head), three sizes straight cross-cut fissure, tapered cross-cut fissure and inverted cone burs (nowadays, rarely used clinically). Burs numbered according to size/diameter of cutting head. Carbon steel heads used for cutting carious dentine but blunt quickly, corrode if not dried after sterilization, now often used as a single-use bur. Similar size carbon steel and TC rose-head burs compared. The TC head is a slightly different shape and is attached to the steel shank. Greater longevity and easily autoclavable. Developments have included the latch-grip, rose-head pattern PKK (polyketone-ketone) plastic bur and other ceramic-based materials **(d)**, for 'self-limiting' carious dentine removal, single-use.

5

Q5.30: What might be the advantages/disadvantages of single-use, disposable burs?

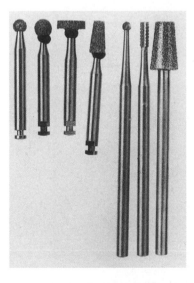

Figure 5.31 A selection of four dental stones mounted on latch-grip short shanks (abrasive carborundum green stones) and three long-shank instruments. Far right is a diamond-coated cone-shaped bur for use in the dental laboratory or rarely at the chairside, for coarse adjustment of indirect restorations and appliances, used at medium speed in a straight handpiece.

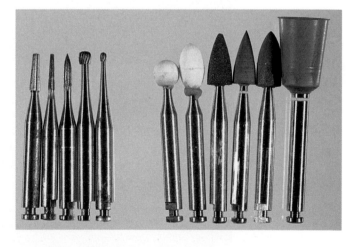

Figure 5.32 Finishing burs, stones, and points for dental amalgam. From the left: five plain-cut latch-grip steel finishing burs, two mounted white (alundum) stones, three mounted abrasive rubber points from coarse to fine, and a mounted abrasive rubber cup.

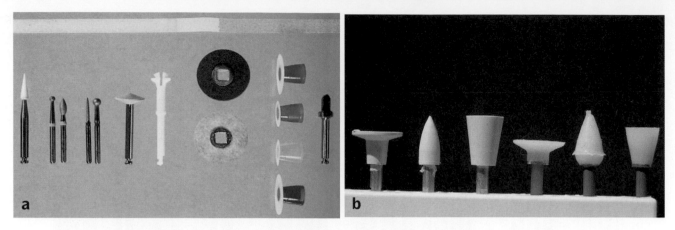

Figure 5.33 (a, b) Composite finishing burs/discs. Across the top is an approximal plastic finishing strip with a blank area in the middle to facilitate passage through the contact point between the teeth. On the right portion the abrasive is coarse and on the left it is fine. From the left: a mounted fine white stone, two medium-grit composite finishing diamonds (yellow band), two fine-grit composite finishing diamonds (red band), a mounted abrasive rubber disc, a mandrel for the two abrasive single-sided flexible discs, which are snap-fit onto the mandrel, and four colour-coded flexible abrasive discs (coarse to fine impregnated grit/diamond) mounted on plastic stubs which fit the mandrel to the right of the picture. In the right image is a series of rubber/resin discs, points and cups impregnated with silica grit enabling the finishing of resin composite and mature glass ionomer cement restorations.

5

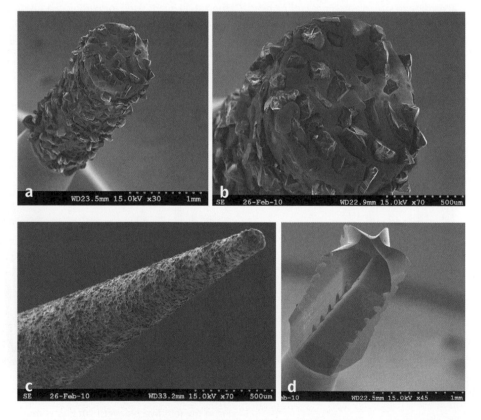

Figure 5.34 (a) Scanning electron micrograph (×30) of a coarse-grit diamond bur. **(b)** same bur as in (a) at 70× magnification showing the random, irregular shapes of the diamond grit. **(c)** 70× magnification of the yellow stripe diamond composite finishing bur with a much smaller grit particle size than the bur in **(a)** or **(b)**. **(d)** 45× magnification of a tungsten carbide Beaver bur used for cutting amalgam and gold – note the sharp notches cut into each flute.

5.8.3 Using hand/rotary instruments – clinical tips

- Rotary instruments cut hard dental tissues by mechanically chipping and smashing away at the ultrastructure of the hard surface. Therefore, the resulting prepared surface is often damaged at the microscopic level (see Figure 5.35). This effect has implications when considering these surfaces as suitable for adhesive bonding (see later).

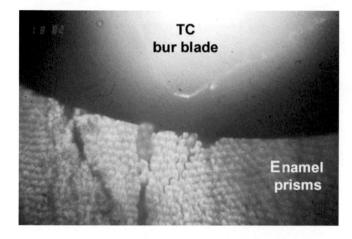

Figure 5.35 Cracks/clefts /cleaving of prisms (horseshoe-shaped structures) after enamel has been cut using a tungsten carbide (TC) bur in an air-turbine handpiece. This inherent damage is unavoidable clinically but can be minimized by using only gentle pressure when operating, copious water spray, and new, sharp burs in a handpiece with sound bearings, allowing vibration-free rotation. The surface and subsurface damage will have implications for adhesive bonding as the shrinkage stresses of adhesive materials exerted on these weakened prisms may open up the cracks further leading to cohesive failure (field width: 200 μm).

- Rotary instruments generate heat at the cutting interface (dissipated by the water spray from both high- and low-speed handpieces), vibration, pressure, and noise (which can deter patients). They provide a reduced tactile feel compared with hand instruments and therefore cutting is guided visually. As a general rule, hard materials (sound enamel, cast metals, and restorations) are cut more efficiently at high speeds and less pressure, whereas softer material (caries) is removed more efficiently at lower speeds and higher torque.

- Water spray ejected from tiny nozzles built into the handpieces should be directed to the tip of the rotating bur head (see Figure 5.28). This cools the tooth surface as it is cut, so preventing excessive frictional heat generation having a deleterious effect on the pulpal tissues. It also helps to flush away debris from the cut tooth surface. The dental nurse should endeavour to keep the mouth mirror free from spray during rotary instrument use, using the 3-1 air/water syringe and aspiration.

- Some handpieces when coupled to the main dental unit enabled with fibreoptics, have the ability to transmit the fibreoptic light from the head of the handpiece directly onto the bur head (see Figure 5.29). This can greatly improve direct vision.

- Air-turbine, rotary burs produce less vibration and pressure. Latch-grip burs have the potential to vibrate.

- The cutting action of rotary (and hand) instrumentation causes a *smear layer* to be formed on cut hard tissue surfaces (usually <50 μm thick). This is a tenacious layer of organic, inorganic, and bacterial debris which is either removed or incorporated in a modified form into the adhesive bond when placing the restoration (see Chapter 6, Section 6.2.4).

- Finger rests: support required for both hand and rotary instrumentation can be achieved by resting the free fingers of the operating hand on a firm structure in the patient's mouth, i.e. adjacent/contralateral/opposing teeth. This provides fine control and reduces risk of iatrogenic damage (see Figures 5.36, 5.37).

- Free hand is used to hold the mouth mirror to provide indirect vision of maxillary arch, reflect light intraorally, and retract soft tissues.

- For the inexperienced operator using rotary instruments, there is a risk of damaging adjacent sound teeth/restorations. As a beginner, it may be wise to protect the adjacent tooth surface with a matrix band.

- With respect to caries removal, burs are not self-limiting and rely on the operator to distinguish between that tissue requiring excavation or not. There has been research into the development of plastic and other non-metallic, single-use burs (see Figure 5.30), which only remove tooth structure that is softer than themselves (anything harder and they will blunt) and so are more self-limiting. Hand excavators rely on the tactile feedback offered to the operator to distinguish the tissue requiring excavation and permit finer discrimination between the carious dentine zones (infected vs. affected vs. sound; see Chapter 1) than rotary instrumentation.

5.8.4 Air-abrasion

- Developed in 1945 by R B Black, air-abrasion is a pseudo-mechanical method for cutting hard dental tissue where the tooth surface is bombarded with high velocity dry abrasive particles in air, transferring kinetic energy to the tooth surface, which is micro-chipped away.

- Adjustable parameters include air pressure, powder flow rate, operating distance, type/size/morphology of the abrasive particle, the diameter of the nozzle tip, and all affect the efficacy and rate of cutting.

- Particles approved by the US Food and Drug Administration (FDA)/or with CE accreditation for clinical use in the mouth include >27 μm alumina and bioactive glass.

- Useful for minimally invasive operative/reparative dentistry with no heat, vibration, pressure, pain or noise generated – rapid operator-dependent tissue removal with alumina particles. The extent of surface/subsurface hard tissue damage (cracks/cleft formation) is far less than using rotary instruments, so making the air-abraded hard surface more conducive to adhesive bonding (see Figure 5.38).

5

5

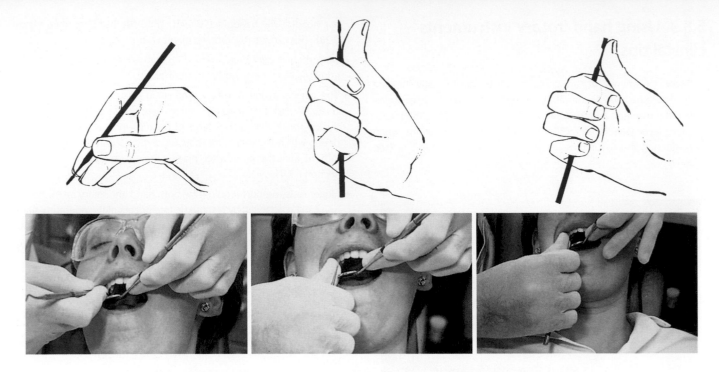

Figure 5.36 From left to right: pen, palm, and finger grip of hand instruments, with clinical examples below. Note how the right hand holding the instrument gains additional finger/thumb support against the patient's adjacent teeth using the remaining free fingers of the operating hand, aiding fine control and reducing the chance of iatrogenic soft/hard tissue damage if the patient suddenly moves their head. Pen grip: most common, most control for fine movement.
Palm/finger grip: limited use for more forceful movements in the maxillary arch. Instrument held between thumb (support) and forefinger with handle across palm, clasped by the remaining fingers.

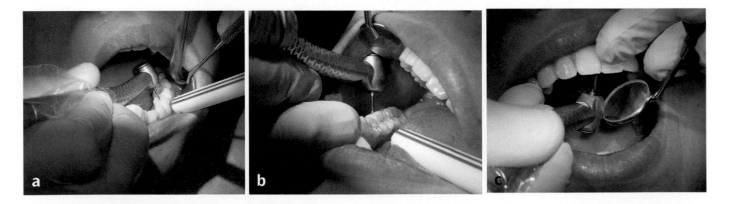

Figure 5.37 Examples of finger rests used by a right-handed dentist while using a dental handpiece. **(a)** Finger rest on the mandibular incisors when operating in the mandibular left quadrant. **(b)** The finger rest on the mandibular right lateral incisor/canine when operating on the mandibular right quadrant. **(c)** Finger rest on the maxillary right canine/premolar region when accessing the maxillary anteriors.

● Bioactive glass particles can be used for extrinsic stain removal, desensitization of exposed cervical dentine, composite removal, and selective demineralized enamel removal (e.g. preventive resin restorations in high caries risk patients, post-orthodontic bracket removal).

● New powders are being investigated for self-limiting carious dentine removal.

● Multi-chambered air-abrasion units allow a metered flow of different particles (alumina, bioactive glass, sodium bicarbonate) in a shroud of water, reducing the dust generated by the process and permitting instantaneous initiation and termination of the abrasive stream (see Figure 5.39); rubber dam is advisable for patient comfort.

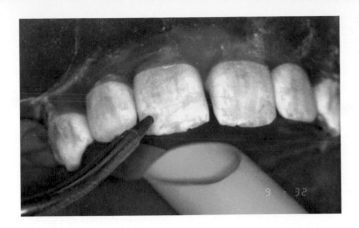

Figure 5.38 An air-abrasion handpiece being used to prepare the labial enamel surfaces of the upper anterior teeth for direct composite veneers. Powder used: dry, 27 μm alumina. Note the blue aspirator tip held close to the operating field to vacuum up the spent powder.

Q5.38: What clinical situations may benefit from using air-abrasion tooth preparation?

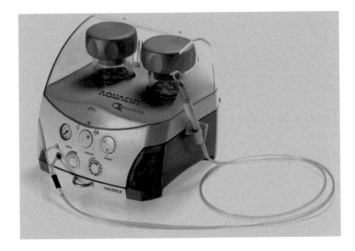

Figure 5.39 An example of a two-chambered dry/wet cutting air-abrasion unit.

5.8.5 Chemo-mechanical methods of caries removal – Carisolv gel

- This is a gel-based dentine caries removal system that reacts with carious dentine that has undergone proteolytic breakdown of collagen, causing further collapse of the collagen network for easy final

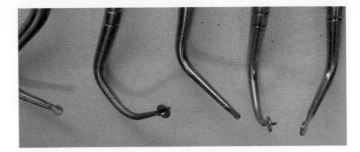

Figure 5.40 A selection of non-cutting, abrasive hand instruments for use with Carisolv gel.

removal with curetting hand instruments. This chemistry confers an element of self-limiting caries removal ability.

- Consists of a 0.1% hypochlorite-based alkaline gel (pH 11) with amino acids preventing breakdown of sound collagen fibrils.

- Stainless steel abrasive, non-cutting hand instruments permit carious dentine removal from cavities (see Figure 5.40). The system requires cavitated lesions for direct access to the carious dentine.

- As excavation is concentrated within caries-affected dentine, patients often do not need local anaesthesia. Gentle hand instrumentation pressure (same force as normal toothbrushing) contributes to reduced patient discomfort (see Figure 5.41).

5.8.6 Other instrumentation technologies

As can be seen from Table 5.5, there are several clinical methods for cutting teeth and removing caries. Ultrasonic and sonic instrumentation use the principle of probe tip oscillation and microcavitation to chip away hard dental tissues. Lasers transfer high energy into the tooth through water causing photoablation of hard tissues. Great control is required by the operator in order to harness this energy effectively and the effects on the remaining enamel, dentine, and pulp are being investigated in terms of residual strength and adhesive bonding capabilities. Enzymatic (including pepsin-based and papain-based) solutions are being investigated to help further breakdown of collagen in already softened carious dentine in the hope of developing a more self-limiting technique of removing caries-infected dentine alone. Other chemical methods include photoactivated disinfection (PAD) – introducing a chemical, tolonium chloride, into the cavity which is taken up by the remaining bacteria in the cavity margins and then activated using light of a specific wavelength, so causing cell lysis and death and ozone (gaseous ozone infused into early lesions causing bacterial death). These technologies currently suffer from a lack of clinical research to validate them for routine evidence-based clinical use.

5

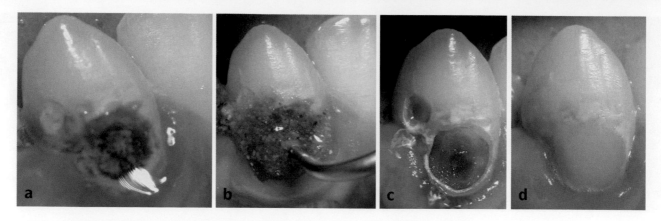

Figure 5.41 Buccal cavitated carious lesion (mICDAS 4) on the LR3. (**a**) Clear Carisolv gel sitting in the cavity for 30 seconds prior to mechanical agitation. (**b**) Gel and carious dentine agitated with a mace tip hand instrument using toothbrushing force. Note how the caries-infected dentine 'emulsifies' into the gel making it cloudy. A repeat application of gel was required in this case to obtain suitable carious dentine removal. No local anaesthetic or rubber dam was required. (**c**) Final cavities before restoration. There has been no direct exposure of the pulp, even though caries excavation is deep. Caries-affected dentine (scratchy but sticky/flaky) has been retained around the gingival margins in this case, along with an intact periphery of enamel (prepared using chisels/gingival margin trimmers (see Figure 5.26). See also Section 5.9. (**d**) Cavity has been restored provisionally with a glass ionomer cement (GIC), during the stabilization stage of the care plan (see Chapter 3).

> Q5.41: Why was the decision taken to retain quantities of caries-affected dentine, especially at the gingival periphery of this particular lesion?

5

5.9 Operative management of the carious lesion

5.9.1 Rationale

The vital aspects of prevention/control of disease and patient management have been discussed in Chapters 3 and 4. There are important factors that will influence the decision to intervene surgically to treat the carious lesion:

- *Aid plaque control*: rough/cavitated tooth surfaces may be difficult for the high risk patient to keep plaque-free (especially in deep occlusal pits/fissures or proximally).

- *The patient's caries risk assessment*: relatively small/early lesions in a high risk patient with poor plaque control may require operative intervention, whereas in a lower risk patient these may require non-operative control (Chapter 4). This is relevant if previous preventive regimens have failed and lesions are progressing.

- *Restore form, function, and appearance*: a large cavitated lesion will weaken the tooth, impeding normal mastication. Smaller, unsightly lesions in the anterior aesthetic zone may require operative intervention, rather than preventive measures alone, for reasons of appearance affecting the patient's inclination to smile and ultimately, their self-confidence.

- *Alleviate pain/'protect' the pulp*: caries removal and a sedative dressing/definitive restoration can remove the symptoms of an acute, reversible pulpitis and allow the dentine–pulp complex to react and heal.

5.9.2 Minimally invasive dentistry

This is part of the overall minimal intervention management philosophy followed in this book – an approach where the dental team bases its individualized patient care on early detection of disease, risk assessment, diagnosis, and prevention/control of further disease with tailored recall appointment frequencies (see Chapters 3 and 8). When operative intervention is required for the above reasons, then the approach should be *minimally invasive*, that is:

1. Excavation of the unrepairable, diseased enamel and dentine only, keeping cavities as small as possible

2. Physically and chemically modifying/optimizing the remaining cavity walls in order to

3. Restore cavities with suitable adhesive materials which will:

   - Support and strengthen the remaining tooth structure

   - Promote remineralization and potentially have antibacterial activity

- Seal off any remaining bacteria from their nutrient supply, so arresting the carious process in the tooth
- Restore appearance and function with suitable long-term success.

In order for this minimally invasive approach to be successful, an integration of your knowledge of histology with the chemistry and handling of dental materials is essential. Also, it is vital that patients understand their responsibility in controlling and preventing further disease progression as discussed in Chapter 4. In modern dental practice, it is imperative that detailed written records are kept highlighting all of the above.

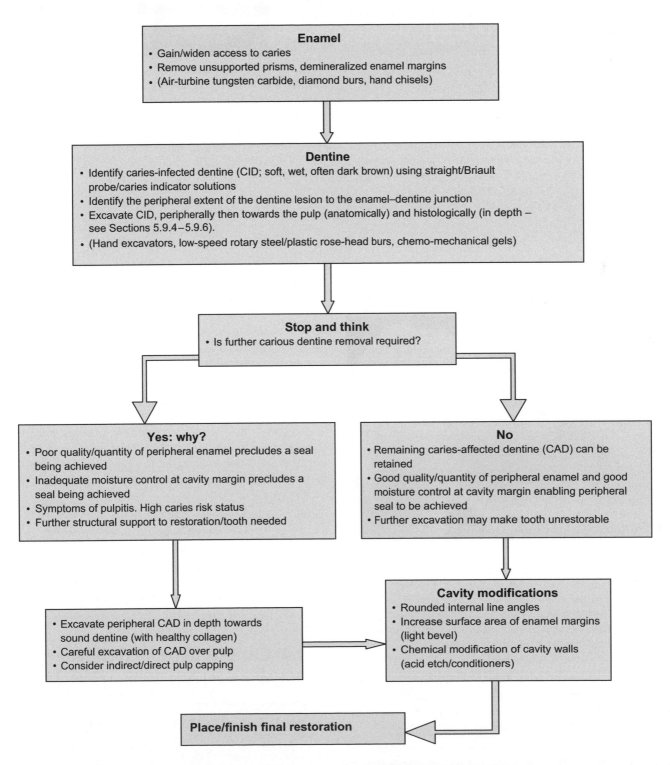

Figure 5.42 Flowchart showing the decision-making process and stages of execution of caries removal following the minimally invasive approach. These stages will be discussed in detail below.

The decision-making process and execution of caries excavation/cavity preparation can be divided into the stages described in the flowchart, Figure 5.42, and will be discussed below.

5.9.3 Enamel preparation

The aims of cutting through enamel when operatively managing a carious lesion are to:

1. Gain visual/instrumentation access to the full extent of the deeper carious dentine requiring removal

2. Remove demineralized, weakened (and often unsightly) carious enamel

3. Create a sound peripheral enamel margin to which an adhesive restorative material can form a seal.

Figure 5.43 shows a histological cross-section through a cavitated, mICDAS 4 lesion with unsupported and demineralized enamel, and the extent of enamel preparation required. These margins may be lightly bevelled to increase the surface area for adhesion. Figure 5.44 shows the clinical occlusal appearance of such enamel removal using a diamond or TC bur in an air-turbine handpiece. This cutting process must be carried out with only gentle pressure avoiding the use of coarse grit diamond burs, so as not to

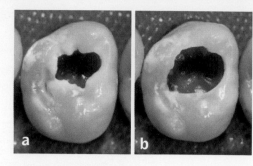

Figure 5.44 An occlusal cavitated carious lesion UR7 (mICDAS 4). **(a)** The lesion at presentation with frosty white demineralized, friable, and unsupported enamel at the cavity margin with carious dentine visible. **(b)** Enamel access has been widened by removal of the weakened peripheral enamel using a diamond bur in an air-turbine handpiece for <10 seconds. The margin has been lightly bevelled.

cause excessive chipping or cracking of the remaining tooth (see Figure 5.35).

Direct visual/instrumentation access to occlusal, buccal, and lingual/palatal carious surfaces is relatively straightforward with good soft tissue retraction and intraoral lighting. Proximal surface lesions (mesial and distal) can be more awkward and approaches here would include:

- Occlusally, accessing initially just medial to the affected marginal ridge and eventually sacrificing it, so creating a proximal box (see Chapter 7).

- Occlusally, accessing medial to the marginal ridge, directing the bur towards the proximal lesion, *tunnelling* beneath the marginal ridge and conserving it. This is only clinically successful if the lesion is sufficiently small and it then might be debated as to whether operative intervention is appropriate! There is also a good chance of fracture of the weakened marginal ridge enamel in service, following restoration.

- Buccal/lingual/palatally, especially if the tooth is rotated and has undergone some gingival recession. Tunnelling from these aspects can result in successful management as long as the lesion is not too extensive, and effective moisture and cavity margin control can be achieved.

- Directly mesial or distal, if the adjacent tooth is missing and space is present to permit direct visual/instrumentation access.

5.9.4 Carious dentine removal

When excavating dentine caries, careful consideration must be given to both:

- 'Anatomical extent' of the lesion, i.e. the lateral extent from the EDJ lesion periphery across to the caries overlying the pulp.

- 'Histological depth' of the lesion, i.e. the collagen and mineral content of caries-infected dentine versus caries-affected dentine versus sound dentine (Chapter 1).

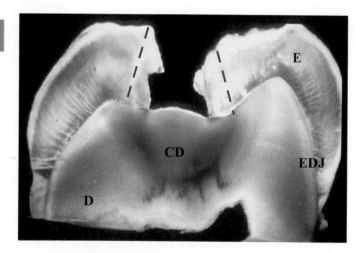

Figure 5.43 A thin mesiodistal longitudinal section through a cavitated lesion (mICDAS 4) viewed in reflected light. Note the demineralized, overhanging enamel bordering the cavity, with the undermining spread of the dentine lesion at the EDJ (see Chapter 1). The red dashed lines indicate the extent of enamel removal required in order to achieve a sound enamel margin with supported prism structure, suitable to affect a seal with an adhesive restorative material while still permitting access to the underlying carious dentine. E, enamel; D, dentine; CD, carious dentine; EDJ, enamel–dentine junction.

Q5.43: What is the name given to the appearance of the alternate light and dark striping evident in the inner third of enamel, arising from the EDJ and radiating towards the tooth surface?

Dentine caries removal must be tailored to the individual lesion, tooth and patient. Following the minimally invasive approach, smaller cavities and restorations are created with the following benefits, ultimately leading to restorations with increased longevity and reduced tissue destruction:

- Adhesive restorative materials are often easier to handle in smaller quantities.

- Moisture control, cavity margin seal, and finish can be better regulated.

- The restored crown is often strengthened due to greater retention of natural, repairable tooth structure.

- Simpler and therefore, improved patient care and maintenance.

5.9.5 Peripheral caries (EDJ)

Prevention of recurrent caries at the margin or caries progression beneath a restoration depends primarily on the seal formed between the restoration and tooth structure at the periphery of the cavity.

- In no clinical situation should caries-infected dentine be retained at the EDJ as this dentine is essentially necrotic and cannot be adhered to.

- The adhesive seal is created optimally between an adhesive restoration and enamel. Therefore, if histologically sound enamel lines the entire periphery of the cavity and moisture control is optimal (e.g. an occlusal cavity), limited brown-discoloured, caries-affected dentine may be retained at the EDJ. This, however, should be selectively removed, down to deeper sound dentine, if there is a risk that the brown discoloration may shine through the restoration, so jeopardizing the final aesthetics.

- If less/no enamel is retained at the EDJ and adequate moisture control cannot be guaranteed (e.g. cervical or proximal lesion, base of a proximal box preparation close to the gingival margin) then sound dentine is a prerequisite at the EDJ in an attempt to maximize the bond and adhesive seal between the retained dentine and final restoration. However, if this means extending the cavity a long way subgingivally, consideration must be given to the long-term success rate of the final restoration and ultimately the final restorability of the tooth in question (see Figure 5.41).

- Distinguishing between caries-infected, affected and sound dentine is a rather subjective skill and the operator usually uses differential tactile judgement (see Table 5.7 below). Brown discoloration of the dentine at the EDJ is neither an indicator of its infectivity nor for its removal (unless in the aesthetic zone).

- Instruments used commonly include hand excavators or steel rose-head burs in a low-speed handpiece. Other technologies might include the chemo-mechanical methods (Table 5.5).

5.9.6 Caries overlying the pulp

When excavating dentine caries overlying the pulp, consideration must be given to its *proximity to the pulp* (see Section 5.11) and any *pulpal symptoms* (see Chapter 3, Section 3.2).

- Where a peripheral seal can be achieved (enamel margins intact) and pulpal symptoms are not present, small quantities of caries-affected dentine may be retained overlying the pulp, so reducing the risk of pulp exposure.

- If the dentine lesion has only penetrated into the middle third of dentine radiographically, thanks to tertiary dentine being laid down at the dentine–pulp border, excavation to sound dentine may be achievable to improve the adhesive bond and seal (especially if enamel margins are not intact).

- Where chronic pulpal symptoms persist along with radiographic changes at the apex, caries excavation needs to be complete, exposing the pulp chamber and its necrotic contents if necessary with a view to the continuation of endodontic treatment.

Table 5.6 summarizes the interlinked factors affecting the decision to remove/retain carious dentine. It must be understood that there is no absolute correct or incorrect amount of caries that should be excavated, but whatever decision is made by the operator, it should be made for sensible, justifiable, and documented reasons. Different amounts of caries can be removed or retained in different parts of the same cavity. Figure 5.45 highlights this variation in dentine caries removal, showing three levels of potential excavation endpoint, depending on the combined outcome of the factors discussed in Table 5.6.

5.9.7 Distinguishing the zones of carious dentine

The clinical discrimination of caries-infected, caries-affected, and sound dentine is at present a subjective skill gained using a combination of an understanding of caries histology with clinical experience. These boundaries are not clearly defined; the histological and bacterial changes occur throughout the whole lesion as a continuum from superficial to deeper layers, with different rates of progression within the individual lesion itself. Table 5.7 summarizes the techniques available, both clinical and through research development, to help enable the operator distinguish these important 'histological' layers. From the table it can be seen that none are truly objective, with interpretation required to decide the excavation endpoint and linked to the factors discussed in Table 5.6.

5.9.8 'Stepwise excavation' and the atraumatic restorative technique (ART)

These two operative techniques are the original and more modern application, respectively, of the minimally invasive approach to managing larger cavitated carious lesions. Both can use simple hand instrumentation (spoon-shaped excavators) to remove the necrotic, superficial layer of caries-infected dentine and some caries-affected dentine also if required (see Figure 5.46). The stages of the original stepwise excavation included the use of a calcium hydroxide lining and a temporary zinc polycarboxylate cement restoration. Between 6 and

5

Table 5.6 A summary of the inter-relating factors affecting the decision of how much dentine caries to excavate (infected vs. affected vs. sound)

Factors affecting amount of carious dentine removed	Comments
Patient's caries risk	High risk, uncontrolled caries progression: earlier lesions may be treated with excavation to sound dentine where possible.
Patient/oral factors	Limited oral opening, physical/mental disability affect visual/instrument access. Broken down/rotated/partially erupted teeth can hinder rubber dam placement. Sedation/general anaesthesia may be required.
Pulp vitality (sensibility)	Chronic symptoms of an irreversible pulpitis will mean pulp extirpation after complete caries removal to sound dentine.
Pulp proximity	If no/limited pulp symptoms, CAD retained over the pulpal depth of cavity to allow remineralization from dentine–pulp complex – indirect pulp capping.
Remaining coronal tooth structure	Sufficient supragingival tooth structure must remain to support the restoration long term. Excavation to sound dentine should not compromise the physical/adhesive properties of the restorative material, e.g. deep peripheral excavation to sound dentine resulting in a cavity margin >2 mm subgingivally, compromising moisture control and marginal adaptation.
Material factors	Retention mechanisms – mechanical, micro-mechanical, chemical adhesion. An adverse oral environment can affect the set and physical properties of some materials, e.g. GICs in xerostomia.

5

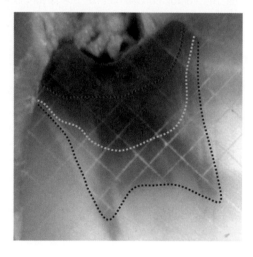

Figure 5.45 A cavitated dentine lesion (mICDAS 3/4) showing the colour gradation from the superficial caries-infected dentine subjacent to the EDJ through to the deeper levels of caries-affected dentine, including the translucent zone and sound dentine. Three positions have been indicated for potential caries excavation endpoints: dark blue dotted line – excavation to sound dentine at EDJ and pulpal aspect; pale blue dotted line – less invasive excavation retaining stained dentine at the EDJ and affected dentine over the pulp; red dotted line – minimally invasive excavation finishing on sound enamel at the EDJ and infected/affected dentine over the pulp. Note how all potential endpoints finish on sound enamel so providing a sealed margin. None of these endpoints are right or wrong, but it is essential that the histology at all levels is appreciated to enable a successful restoration to be placed.

Q5.45: Which of the three positions do you think would be best to stop caries removal, in the above lesion?

9 months later, this restoration was removed, exposing the remaining, now arrested caries-affected dentine (darker, harder, and dryer) and deposited tertiary dentine. The stained dentine was removed using a steel rose-head bur in a low-speed handpiece and a final amalgam restoration placed. The more recently developed ART proposes restoring the cavity with chemically adhesive, high-viscosity GIC, forming a better adaptive seal to the remaining tooth structure (see Chapter 6) following the use of simple hand excavators to gain access to and remove the caries-infected dentine. This restoration does not necessarily require complete replacement as the arrested caries-affected dentine is sealed off from its nutrient supply. However, occlusal resurfacing of the GIC may be necessary after 2–3 years due to wear and partial dissolution. This can be accomplished with a layer of composite on the surface of the GIC – an *adhesive layered*, *laminate* or 'sandwich' restoration (see Chapter 7).

Both stepwise excavation and ART follow the principles of minimally invasive dentistry. As this is an accepted rationale for operative caries management, these terminologies are now rather redundant as current adhesive dental materials are more capable of sealing in and potentially rehabilitating diseased tissue.

Table 5.7 Clinical and research methods used to help clinically discriminate between the three histological zones of carious dentine (infected, affected, and sound). Note that these zones do not have distinct boundaries but have a gradient of histological/bacterial change through them from the enamel–dentine junction (EDJ) to the pulp (see Chapter 1)

Discriminating methods		Caries-infected dentine	Caries-affected dentine	Sound dentine
Clinical	*Visual*	Often a colour gradient from (Figure 5.45): Dark brown → paler brown/translucent → yellow/white Very difficult to judge clinically/OK when examining a sectioned lesion (research).		
	Tactile	Soft/sticky feel with a sharp dental probe (straight or Briault).	Both sticky/flaky and scratchy feel.	Scratchy feel to a sharp dental probe.
	Caries detector dyes	'Fusayama' dyes – based on propylene-glycol, collagen-based stain. Attempts to discriminate infected versus affected but research has shown these dyes stain deeper collagen in affected/sound dentine zones often leading to cavity over-preparation.		
Research development	*Bacterial dyes*	Dyes under research development reacting to bacterial redox byproducts – using their concentration gradient drop from infected through affected to sound dentine. Has potential to be zone-selective.		
	Fluorescence	Research into the natural fluorescence of dentine caries using confocal fibreoptic microendoscopy indicates a discriminating level of fluorescence of infected dentine. A technique that might be developed for *in vivo* use in the future.		

5

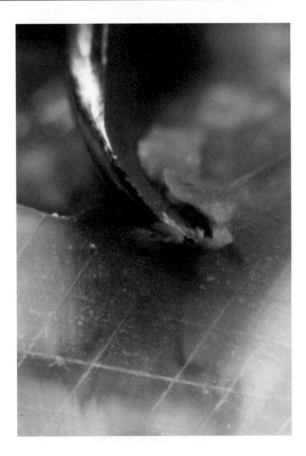

Figure 5.46 Hand excavator scooping through necrotic, soft caries-infected dentine once the enamel access has been widened (reference grid lines on the dentine face were placed for measuring purposes).

5.10 Cavity modification

Once caries removal is complete, the dentist needs to stop, think and decide which restorative material to use and then modify the cavity accordingly (Figure 5.47), if required. These changes may be necessary to improve the retentive properties or to maximize the material properties, e.g. bulk strength or fracture resistance.

- *Retention*: the property of a cavity that resists displacement of the restoration in the direction of its insertion.

- *Cavity support*: the cavity property that prevents displacement (or fracture) of the restoration in any other direction, including internal dislodgement within the cavity itself. This feature relates to the morphology of cavity walls/floors and rounded internal line angles.

Table 5.8 outlines the different macro- (bur-induced) or micro-modifications (chemically induced) dependent on the restorative material to be used.

Table 5.8 Potential cavity modifications required after caries removal, depending on the material chosen to restore the cavity*

Restorative material	Cavity modification		Comments
Composite/GIC	macro	Enamel margin bevel (short/long)	Removes grossly unsupported prisms. Increases surface area for bond/seal. Provides a sound enamel surface to facilitate optimal adhesive bonding (Figures 5.43, 5.44).
All	macro	Rounded internal line angles	Reduces both internal stresses and risk of crack propagation within the restoration (Figures 5.48, 5.50, 5.51).
Composite	micro	Enamel acid etch	37% orthophosphoric acid removes smear layer, selectively demineralizes prisms creating micro-mechanical undercuts for resin retention.
GIC	micro	Dentine conditioner	10% polyacrylic/citric acids, modify or remove smear layer, preparing the surface for chemical adhesion (Ca^{2+}).
Amalgam	macro	Cavity undercuts, grooves, slots, flat surfaces	Cavities with wider bases than orifices are required for retention of amalgam – undercuts. Slots/grooves help prevent further displacement of the restoration (Figures 5.49, 5.50). Flat cavity surfaces with rounded internal line angles help improve the cavity support (Figure 5.51).
All	macro	Pulp chamber	In endodontically treated teeth, the pulp chamber is used to add bulk and retentive features/increased surface area for the coronal restoration.
Amalgam	macro	Nayyar core	Packing the coronally flared 2–3 mm of endodontically treated root canals to improve core retention.
Gold, porcelain, composite (indirect restorations)	macro	Long marginal taper	Divergent tapered margins (7–10°) used to improve retentive features of indirect restorations.

* The modifications have been classified as macro (those created using a bur) or micro (those created using chemicals). See Chapter 6 for a description of the material science and Chapter 7 for practical considerations.

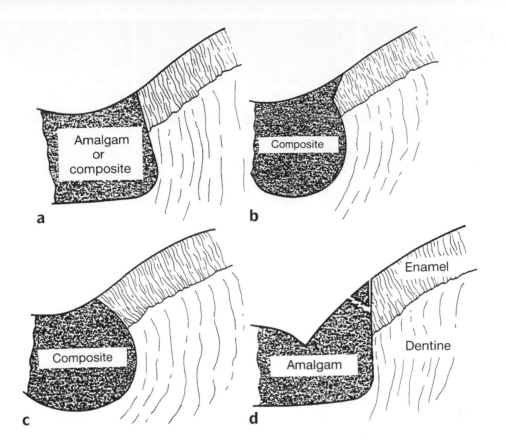

Figure 5.47 Diagrams outlining the different restoration margin angles and cavosurface angles that are suited to different restorative materials. (**a**) Amalgam and composite margins require bulk for strength so 90° restoration margin angles and cavosurface angles will ensure sufficient intrinsic strength of both the restoration margin and cavity edge. (**b**) Resin composites adhere and support enamel to a degree so light bevelling of the enamel surface can increase the surface area for adhesive bonding while also removing any potentially unsupported enamel prisms at the cavity edge (**c**). (**d**) If the amalgam margin angle is too acute, the amalgam margin may be weakened sufficiently for marginal fracture to occur under occlusal loading.

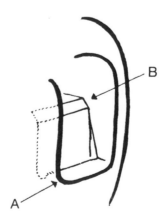

Figure 5.48 Diagram indicating the internal bevelling/rounding off of the internal line angles between adjacent internal cavity surfaces (A and B). This reduces the risk of crack propagation within the restorative material.

5

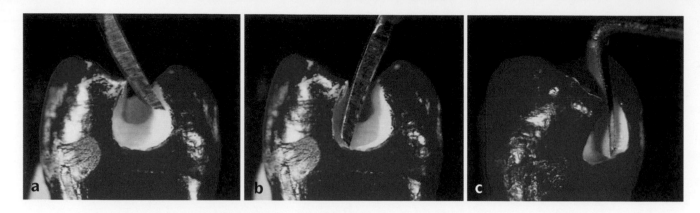

Figure 5.49 (a–c) Approximal box cavities prepared with undercuts (a wider base and a narrower occlusal opening) to prevent displacement of the restoration (amalgam) occlusally, from its path of insertion.

Q5.49: Which hand instrument is shown in Figure 5.49

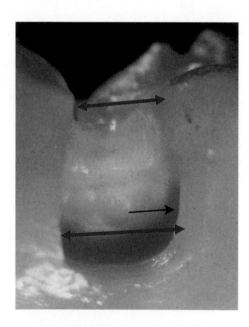

Figure 5.50 An approximal box cavity prepared with occlusal undercuts (wider base, narrow occlusal opening – red arrows) to prevent displacement of the restoration (amalgam) from its path of insertion occlusally. Note the rounded internal line angles. The black arrow shows the placement of a groove at the junction between the buccal wall of the box and the pulpal wall, so providing resistance to proximal displacement.

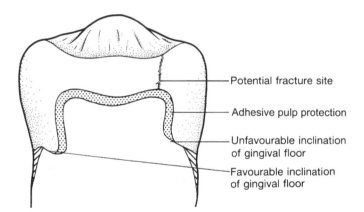

Potential fracture site

Adhesive pulp protection

Unfavourable inclination of gingival floor

Favourable inclination of gingival floor

Figure 5.51 Potential problems of the morphology of cavity walls and floor, requiring modification. Rounded internal line angles reduce the risk of crack propagation and eventual restoration fracture of rigid materials (e.g. amalgam). Use of a rose-head bur to remove carious dentine tends to create the cavity floor morphology on the left but care must be taken to remove any very prominent unsupported enamel lip at the periphery. The floor morphology on the right offers limited support to the final restoration and should be avoided.

5.11 Pulp protection

5.11.1 Rationale

The final consideration along with any cavity modifications, prior to placing the restoration, is the long-term pulp status. This is linked to *pulpal signs and symptoms* and *cavity proximity* to the pulp. Assuming the symptoms and signs of pulp sensibility indicate a histologically viable pulp (see Chapter 3), the pulpal tissues may require protection from:

- Bacteria/toxins
- Chemicals leaching from the restorative materials (e.g. unconverted resin monomers)
- Thermal and/or electrical stimulation via conductance through the overlying restoration.

If the floor of the cavity is close to the pulp but the pulp chamber has not been breached during caries removal, then this protection can be afforded by a process termed *indirect pulp capping (IPC)*. If a small breach, or *pulp exposure*, has occurred (usually no wider than the tip of a Williams periodontal probe), created either iatrogenically or by the carious process, a *direct pulp cap (DPC)* may be placed in an attempt to maintain pulp viability but the patient must be warned that this is not guaranteed, especially when this is a consequence of a deep carious cavity.

5.11.2 Terminology

There are two older terms used in the dental literature to describe this form of material-based pulp protection where an exposure has not occurred: *cavity lining* and *structural base*. These terms were coined when amalgam was the only material of choice to restore cavities long term and it was thought the pulp required an 'insulating' layer between it and the metal-based restoration. The often excessively large, undercut cavities designed for amalgam could be artificially reduced in size by placing zinc oxide-based plastic materials as 'structural bases', on to which was packed a reduced volume of amalgam. The authors believe that in the modern era of minimally invasive dentistry, these terms should no longer be used so as to avoid further confusion.

5.11.3 Materials

Materials used for both IPC and DPC should ideally:

- Be bactericidal/static

- Be mildly irritant to the pulp to stimulate tertiary dentine bridge formation (usually via pH changes)
- Be adhesive in order to affect a bond and seal
- Not dissolve away over time
- Be strong and easily applied in thin section
- Be able to infiltrate ionically into the remaining dentine overlying the pulp, so strengthening/reinforcing it
- Be biocompatible with the pulp and overlying restorative material.

Clinical dental materials used for IPC/DPC (see Chapter 6) include:

- GIC lining materials
- Dentine bonding agents
- Setting calcium hydroxide materials
- Mineralized trioxide aggregate (MTA) and derivatives.

The first two materials fulfil the majority of the above criteria of an ideal IPC. When using these adhesive materials as the final restorative solution, it may be argued that a separate thin layer of pulp protection may not be necessary as the properties are 'built in' to the bulk restorative material itself. Calcium hydroxide cements have been used for many years as pulp protection beneath amalgam restorations but in recent times, much more sparingly. The authors cannot suggest any positive indications for their use beneath adhesive restorations as an IPC. GICs and resin-based cements are being used more often for bonded amalgam restorations, so again, the use of calcium hydroxide is ever more limited in this regard. As a DPC, the alkaline pH of calcium hydroxide still has a use as an inflammatory stimulant for pulpal odontoblasts to produce tertiary dentine and close the exposure. Unset MTA is primarily calcium oxide in the form of tricalcium silicate, dicalcium silicate, and tricalcium aluminate, with bismuth oxide added for radio-opacity. Several studies indicate its potential use as a DPC as it increases the concentration of available calcium hydroxide, the primary reaction product between MTA and water, and provides a seal. Both setting calcium hydroxide cements and slow-setting MTA may need a second protective covering prior to placing the final restoration. A faster setting, stronger MTA derivative 'Biodentine' has recently been introduced as a dentine replacement restorative material. This is conventionally a GIC/resin-modified (RM)-GIC material (Chapter 6).

5.12 Dental matrices (see also Chapter 7)

Cavities created with missing proximal walls provide a technical problem when it comes to placing a direct plastic restorative material, as there is nothing to contain the restoration within the cavity or to prevent poor marginal adaptation (ledges, overhangs). *Circumferential* (e.g. reusable Siqveland and Tofflemire; disposable Automatrix and Omni-matrix; see Figure 5.52) or *sectional* matrix bands have been

developed to rectify this problem (Palodent, Composi-Tight, V-Ring, Quickmat). Dental matrices consist of two components:

- *Single-use matrix band*: thin metal or clear plastic band of varying widths and gauges (30–50 μm) used to form the missing wall of the cavity. More rigid and wider bands used posteriorly

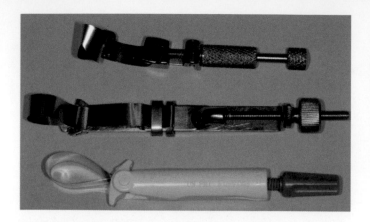

Figure 5.52 Three circumferential metal matrix bands with retainers. Top: Tofflemire retainer with precurved matrix band; middle: Siqveland retainer with matrix band; bottom: Omni-matrix disposable system.

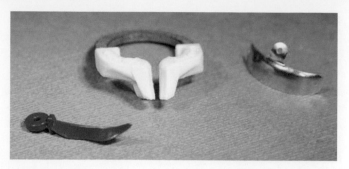

Figure 5.53 A precurved and contoured single-use sectional metal matrix band (right) with a plastic gingivally contoured wedge (left) and the oval ring retainer with curved tines (middle) to adapt the band to the approximal surface of the tooth. The retainer can be sterilized.

(metal) and narrower pliable plastic bands used anteriorly (for composites).

- *Retainer*: a device used to tighten and hold circumferential matrix bands in place proximally. These can be sterilized and used again. Sectional matrix systems have oval/round ring retainers with curved tines to adapt the matrix to the proximal tooth contour (see Figure 5.53).

5.12.1 Clinical tips

- Cervical margin adaptation of the band to the tooth is essential to prevent ledges or overhangs of excess restorative material, often requiring the use of wooden/plastic wedges in the interproximal space.

- Tight interdental contact points may need to be slightly opened by causing differential movement of the adjacent teeth within their periodontal ligament spaces. This is accomplished by prewedging using wooden wedges for a few minutes prior to placing the band.

- Sectional matrices may be of benefit in situations where teeth are rotated or tilted so making the placement of circumferential bands more difficult.

- Sectional bands are more adaptable to gain well-contoured proximal surfaces and contact areas.

- Circumferential bands can be more painful for the patient to endure than equivalent sectional bands.

- Clear plastic bands/wedges can be used when placing composite restorations to permit light penetration to the depths of the proximal cavity when curing the material.

- Rubber dam clamps may have to be removed prior to placing matrix bands.

- Anteriorly, if contact areas are tight and the flexible, clear plastic matrix band refuses to pass through incisally, the corner of the band can be cut to a point and passed cervically beneath the contact and then lifted incisally through it.

5.13 Temporary (intermediate) restorations

5.13.1 Definitions

Temporary restoration is one that is placed for short-term use (usually days or weeks) often between appointments in a course of ongoing definitive treatment (e.g. caries stabilization, multivisit root canal treatment, simple fixed prosthodontics).

Provisional restoration is one that is placed for short/medium-term duration (weeks/months) where diagnostic value is gained from placing the restoration (e.g. complex fixed prosthodontic treatment when reorganizing a patient's occlusion or adjusting the vertical dimension of the patient's occlusion (see later)).

The dental material science of temporary restorations (GIC, zinc oxide eugenol, and zinc polycarboxylates) is covered in Chapter 6. Eugenol-containing temporary restorations should be avoided in cavities where the final restoration to be placed is a resin composite, as the eugenol affects the polymerization chemistry.

5.13.2 Clinical tips

- Care must be taken when placing temporary restorations to replicate the occlusion and marginal adaptation of the restoration.

- Zinc oxide-based materials have a relatively poor appearance, so, in the anterior aesthetic zone, GIC-based materials might be considered.

- Patients must be made fully aware of the reason and function of the temporary restoration.
- Adequate time must be allocated in the clinical appointment to place temporary restorations. Poor quality marginal adaptation of

temporaries can lead to further marginal staining, plaque accumulation and gingival inflammation/bleeding, which in turn often worsens the patients' oral hygiene procedures.

5.14 Principles of dental occlusion

In order to successfully restore dental function in the long term, an understanding of human dental occlusion is of primary importance. This subject is complex and many textbooks exist discussing these complexities and their clinical relevance. The occlusal contacts between the maxillary and mandibular dentition are affected by the skeletal base relationship (condylar head vs. slope of the articular eminence, glenoid fossa), development of the maxilla and mandible, and direct factors affecting the development, position, and shape of the teeth themselves. Analysis of occlusion is critical in both the *conformative* or *reorganizational* approaches to managing dental care.

5.14.1 Definitions

Conformative approach An approach to planning and placing restorations that ensures the pre-existing occlusal relationships are not altered in any of the three planes (anteroposterior, vertical, and horizontal). It is essential therefore to analyse aspects of the occlusion prior to commencing so the final restorations fit into the existing scheme. This approach most often applies when placing single or multiple plastic, direct restorations.

Re-organized approach This approach involves changes in occlusion and is often undertaken when rehabilitating major occlusal discrepancies caused by tilting or over-eruption of teeth resulting in premature occlusal interference contacts and/or distortion of the occlusal planes causing reduced space into which to place definitive restorations. Here again, considerable planning with the use of provisional restorations is required in order to calculate the tolerances of changing the occlusion. This approach is usually indicated in complex cases often involving the use of indirect restorations (crowns, bridges, dentures, or implants) and is outwith the scope of this textbook.

5.14.2 Terminology

The commonly used terminology and recorded positions of occlusal analysis are described in Table 5.9.

5

Table 5.9 Various occlusal relationships, their definitions, and relevance to restorative dentistry

Occlusal relationship	Definition	Diagram/comments
Intercuspal position (ICP) (static)	The occlusal relationship where there is maximum cuspal interdigitation between the maxillary and mandibular teeth.	Not always clinically reproducible and can be affected by occlusal interferences.
Occlusal vertical dimension (OVD) (static)	The vertical relationship between the maxilla and mandible with the teeth in ICP.	Can be reduced by toothwear, missing teeth. Can be compensated biologically by over-eruption of teeth/dento-alveolar compensation.
Rest position (RP)/resting vertical dimension (RVD) (static)	The vertical relationship between the maxilla and mandible when resting comfortably in an upright position with relaxed facial musculature.	Achieved after swallowing/yawning. Teeth usually slightly apart.
Freeway space (FS) (static)	The vertical dimension difference between RP and OVD (ranges 2–4 mm).	Adaptive in the dentate patient. Essential consideration for the restoration of the edentate individual with complete dentures.

(Continued)

Occlusal relationship	Definition	Diagram/comments
Overjet (OJ) (static)	The horizontal distance between the maxillary and mandibular incisal edges in ICP.	Overjet
Overbite (OB) (static)	The vertical distance between the maxillary and mandibular incisal edges in ICP. No vertical overlap can lead to an edge-edge incisal relationship or an anterior open bite (AOB).	Overbite
Retruded contact position (RCP) (dynamic)	The most retruded position of the mandible when there is initial cuspal contact (described as the relationship where the condylar heads are rearmost within their glenoid fossae and rotate about their terminal hinge axis or *centric relation*).	A clinically reproducible and registerable position used in the dental rehabilitation of the edentulous patient as well as in the reorganized approach in the dentate patient.
Lateral excursions (dynamic)	Occlusal relationship between the teeth when the mandible is shifted horizontally to the right or left. Working side: the side to which the mandible has moved. Non-working side: the side away from which the mandible has moved.	Horizontal movement guided by working side: 1. Palatal/labial surfaces of canines/incisors. 2. Cuspal inclines of premolars/molars. 3. A combination of both. Horizontal movement may also be guided by non-working side contacts and condylar head–glenoid fossae relationships.
Protrusion (dynamic)	The anterior/forward movement of the mandible with teeth in occlusion.	Usually guided by the palatal contour of the maxillary incisors. Leads to a posterior open bite – Christensen's phenomenon.

5.14.2 Occlusal registration techniques

The various static and dynamic relationships of the patient's occlusion should be analysed before starting any restorative procedure in the conformative approach of dental care provision, as well as checking again after the restoration(s) has been completed. There are many different clinical techniques available for checking direct occlusal contact relationships in the patient's mouth:

- *Articulating paper*: ranges 40–200 μm in thickness, different colours that show up contact areas between cusp inclines and fossae on occlusion (Figure 5.54).

- *Shimstock*: articulating foil (8 μm) for the fine occlusal adjustment of coronal restorations.
- *Clinical observation*: assess dental contacts around the arch prior to removing an old/damaged restoration and ensure these are replicated with the new restoration, especially in the partially dentate.

5.14.4 Clinical tips

- Occlusion must be checked both *before* and *after* placement of any restoration affecting the occlusal or guidance surfaces of teeth. Different colour articulating paper can be used in this regard. This is essential in the conformative approach to dental care provision.

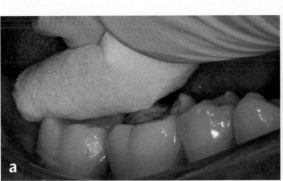
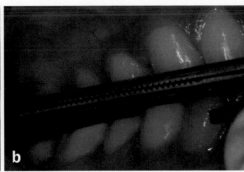
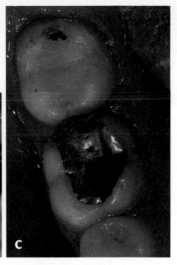

Figure 5.54 (a) Occlusal surfaces of LR quadrant being dried with a cotton wool roll. (b) Articulating paper held in forceps placed on occlusal surfaces and patient asked to bite together in the intercuspal position (ICP) and slide teeth left and right. (c) Heavy occlusal cusp–fossa contact shown on distal occlusal aspect of LR7 (red mark – ICP, black – lateral excursions). This can now be selectively removed with a rotary instrument.

Q5.54a: Why is it important to dry the teeth prior to using dental articulating paper?

Q5.54b: What mandibular movements should the patient be encouraged to make when checking the occlusion using articulating paper?

- Occlusal surfaces should be dried with cotton wool rolls (see Figure 5.54a).
- Occlusion must be checked dynamically as well as statically. Patients must be asked to 'grind' their teeth side to side and back to front in order to check the guidance paths are free from interferences.

- Even though some authorities classify the buccal cusps of the mandibular teeth and palatal cusps of the maxillary dentition as *functional cusps*, it must be realized that all cusps, ridges, and fossae have an important role to play in a harmonious dynamic occlusion.

5

5.15 Answers to self-test questions

Q5.8: Can you spot the gold crown?

A: It is present on the upper right hand side of the radiograph – the discrete radio-opacity.

Q5.18: Can you spot a clinical omission in Figure 5.18?

A: The safety floss around the connector arm and through the holes of the clamp is missing. This aids in retrieving pieces in cases of clamp separation.

Q5.22: In which clinical situations might you use each of the probes above?

A: Straight probe – clinical examination of restoration margins and exposed carious dentine; Briault probe – proximal surfaces, internal cavity walls; Williams probe – periodontal pocket assessment, clinical exam of tooth surfaces; Naber's probe – periodontal furcation measurement; CPITN probe – periodontal assessment, clinical examination of tooth surfaces.

Q5.25: What are the advantages of having angulations between the working heads and shanks of these instruments?

A: To enable the operator to access all aspects of a cavity, undercut, or undermined areas as well as off-setting the handle to allow better direct visual access to instrumentation.

Q5.30: What might be the advantages/disadvantages of single-use, disposable burs?

A: Advantages – improved infection control, no maintenance required; disadvantages – potential long-term cost, possible concerns about quality control over the precision in manufacture, availability of all types of bur.

Q5.38: What clinical situations may benefit from using air-abrasion tooth preparation?

A: Minimally invasive dentistry procedures – diagnosing and treating carious fissures in high risk patients with unmodifiable risk factors, tooth preparation for direct labial composite veneers, all tooth surface pre-treatment prior to adhesive bonding, stain removal/refreshing surfaces of old composites, potential selective enamel/dentine caries removal (with bioactive glass particles – in development).

Q5.41: Why was the decision taken to retain quantities of caries-affected dentine, especially at the gingival periphery of this particular lesion?

A: This was a conscious decision as an intact enamel periphery was present to create an adhesive seal. If the carious dentine was removed at the EDJ (as normal) this would result in a cavity margin that would be located on root dentine at least 3–4 mm subgingivally, with no enamel present. Moisture control would then be impossible, no seal achievable, and the tooth/cavity would be unrestorable. By retaining this affected dentine, the tooth (dentine–pulp complex) has been given the opportunity to heal itself, with suitable input from the patient as regards to oral hygiene and dietary concerns.

Q5.43: What is the name given to the appearance of the alternate light and dark striping evident in the inner third of enamel, arising from the EDJ and radiating towards the tooth surface?

A: Hunter–Schreger bands.

Q5.45: Which of the three positions do you think would be best to stop caries removal, in the above lesion?

A: Probably the second level (pale blue dotted line) on caries-affected dentine where the collagen has partial structure to enable some form of dentine bonding to take place and the periphery histological status will allow a seal to be achieved, while not encroaching on the pulp and risking exposure.

Q5.49: Which hand instrument is shown in Figure 5.49?

A: Gingival margin trimmer.

Q5.54a: Why is it important to dry the teeth prior to using dental articulating paper?

A: To allow the ink from the paper to adhere to and mark the teeth in discrete areas of tooth–tooth contact.

Q5.54b: What mandibular movements should the patient be encouraged to make when checking the occlusion using articulating paper?

A: Vertical intercuspal position (patient should bite up and down) and also lateral excursions (patient should be asked to grind their teeth side to side to assess the cuspal inclines guiding the occlusion in these directions).

6

Restorative materials and their relationship with tooth structure

Chapter contents

6.1 Introduction

Modern restorative materials can be classified in several ways, in terms of their retention (chemically adhesive, macro-, micro- or even nano-mechanical), their chemistry (e.g. resin-based vs. siloxane-oxirane vs. acid–base reaction, filler particles), or their clinical properties (e.g. aesthetics, strength, handling). It is essential that these materials are considered closely with the histological substrate to which they will adhere/interact, in order to understand the complexities of each system and their potential clinical uses.

This chapter will outline and discuss aspects of dental materials science to enable the reader to understand and appreciate the links with relevant histology and relate this to the clinical aspects of operative dentistry. Also discussed is dental amalgam, still a popular restorative material among many dentists but clinical indications for its use are becoming more limited as treatment rationales change and adhesive materials improve. This text will require supplementation from suitable dental histology and dental material science texts.

6.2 Dental composite

Dental resin composites are aesthetic, plastic restorative materials that consist of co-polymerized methacrylate-based resin chains embedding inert filler particles (conferring strength and wear resistance) and requiring a separate adhesive (bonding agent) to micro-/nano-mechanically bond them to either enamel or dentine, respectively. However, not all modern dental composites are purely based on this methacrylate resin chemistry (see Section 6.2.6). Therefore, the terminology 'composite resin' is now inappropriate and should not be used.

6.2.1 History

Composites have developed over the past 50 years, after the introduction of the acid-etch technique (Buonocore, 1955) and methacrylate monomers (Bowen's resin – Bis-GMA (1961), see below).

6.2.2 Chemistry

Methacrylate resins

The unset (or uncured) material consists of a mixture of several different types of resin methacrylate monomers, most of which are hydrophobic (water-hating) in nature (see Figure 6.1).

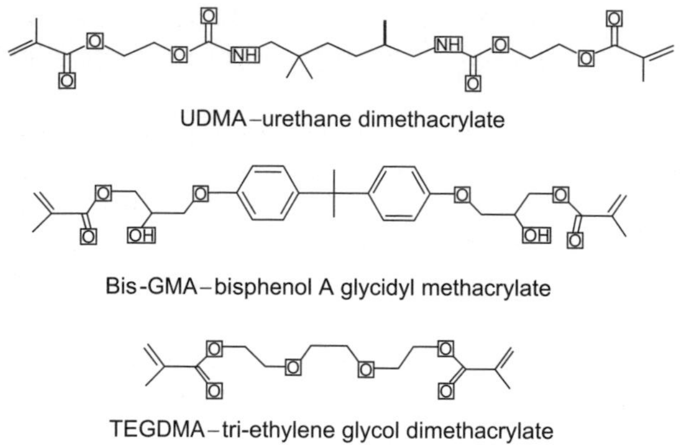

UDMA – urethane dimethacrylate

Bis-GMA – bisphenol A glycidyl methacrylate

TEGDMA – tri-ethylene glycol dimethacrylate

Figure 6.1 Examples with chemical formulae of commonly used methacrylate resins in dental composites. Note how TEGDMA has a shorter chain length than the others.

Q6.1: What properties of the dental composite does monomer chain length affect?

The monomer chain length affects certain properties of the resin composite:

- *Viscosity (or flowability) of the material*: this is important in order to minimize voids trapped within the uncured composite during placement and packing within the depths of a cavity (the stiffer the consistency, the greater the risk of trapping air voids). The shorter the monomer chain length (and therefore, the molecular weight), the less is the viscosity. Often shorter length, lower molecular weight

methacrylate monomers form the basis of the resin chemistry of flowable composites, and other diluent molecules may be added.

- *Volumetric polymerization shrinkage of composite on curing*: the setting process is a light-activated, addition free-radical polymerization chain reaction. The shorter the monomer chains, the more of them need to join per unit volume and the increased reduction in space between them leads to the shrinkage exhibited (1.5–3.5%vol; Figure 6.2)

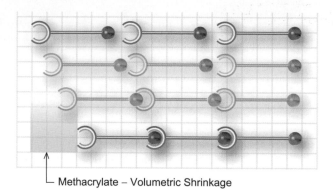

Methacrylate – Volumetric Shrinkage

Figure 6.2 A diagrammatic representation of linear monomers undergoing addition polymerization leading to volumetric shrinkage. (Courtesy of 3MESPE.)

Filler particles (see Figure 6.3)

Inert filler particles are made from silica, quartz, barium, or strontium glass derivatives (so introducing radio-opacity) and are embedded in and bound to the resin matrix using a coating of an organo-silane coupling agent (γ-methacryloxypropyltrimethoxysilane (γ-MPTS)). Over the past 40 years, manufacturers have tried to pack in various sizes/shapes of particle in increasing numbers per unit volume in an effort to adapt the clinical properties of dental composites. The more space taken up by irregular and spherical-shaped filler particles, the less there is for native resin monomer, leading to a reduction in overall shrinkage on curing. Conversely, the more filler particles loaded into the composite, the more viscous it becomes so there is a fine line between balancing the filler load and its resin content. The filler particles confer several properties on the cured composite material:

- *Wear characteristics*: increasing the density of larger, harder and more irregularly shaped filler particles will tend to increase the wear resistance of the composite as less resin matrix will be exposed at the surface.

- *Surface polishability*: the smaller, softer and more spherical-shaped the filler particles, the more polishable the composite (but less wear resistant).

- *Aesthetics*: the finer the filler particles, the more aesthetic the composite as the optical properties can be made to match more accurately that of enamel. Modern composites can have numerous shades (using pigments) or just a few, relying on a 'chameleon' effect where one shade of composite can encompass several tooth shades, blending into the surrounding natural colours very effectively.

6

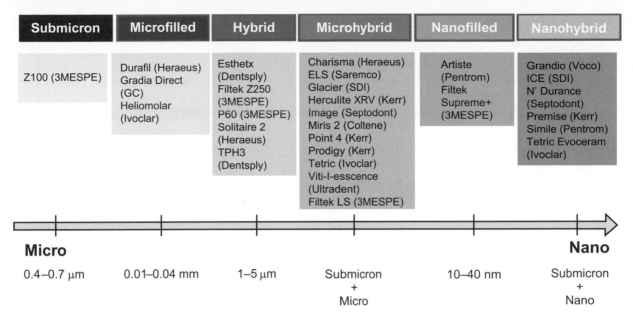

Figure 6.3 A diagram showing the size ranges of filler particles in a range of modern dental resin composites and their manufacturers. (Courtesy of Septodont UK.)

- *Physical properties, e.g. compressive and shear strength, elasticity*: the correct balance of filler particle:resin content is required to ensure optimal physical properties.

Other chemical ingredients

These small fractions include *inhibitors* (butyl-4-hydroxytoluenes (BHT)) to increase material longevity prior to curing, *photo-initiators* (see below), *accelerators* (dimethylaminobenzoates (DMAB), increasing the reactivity of the photo-initiator so speeding up curing time), *photo-stabilizers* (2-hydroxy-4-methoxybenzophenone (HMBP), providing colour stability by eliminating UV action on amine initiators), *opacifiers* (aluminium, titanium or zirconium oxides), and *colour pigments* (various ferric and titanium oxides).

Setting reaction

The setting (curing) process in modern composites is commonly light-activated (470 nm wavelength visible blue light) or dual-cured, light and chemical activation (initiated by 0.5% benzoyl peroxide and activated using dimethyl-p-toluidine). Light-cured composite contains a photo-initiator, α-diketone (camphorquinone) and an amine, which under the activation of the blue light generates the free radicals to initiate the cross-linking polymerization chain reaction. Some issues related to the setting reaction of resins include:

- *Low degree of monomer conversion (50–67%)*: not all the free monomer polymerizes on curing leaving some to leach out of the composite so contributing to the long-term degradation of the material in terms of moisture ingress and possible sensitization issues with some patients.

- *High linear/volumetric shrinkage on curing (1.5–3.5%)*: Figure 6.2 illustrates how shrinkage occurs during polymerization and leads to the composite pulling away from cavity margins so increasing the risk of marginal leakage.

- *High shrinkage stress at the composite–tooth interface (3–8 MPa)*: the stresses generated by the polymerization process can be high at cavity margins (depending on the cavity C-factor (the ratio of bonded vs. unbonded surfaces), the bulk of the material and the compliance of the cavity walls). This can lead to debonding and tooth fracture of the weakened marginal tissues.

- *Water absorption*: water is absorbed hygroscopically during and after the curing process leading to expansion, long-term composite degradation, and staining.

- *Air-inhibited surface layer of uncured resin*: the free radical addition polymerization reaction is inhibited by air. After curing an increment of composite material, a glossy film of uncured resin is retained on the surface of the composite and the monomers in this layer are used to provide adherence for the next increment of composite placed upon it. In this way, composite material can be added to within a cavity to build up the final restoration.

- *Depth of cure*: conventional composites can be cured to a depth of 2–3 mm (depending on the translucency of the material). A thicker section will not cure sufficiently at its base (the 470 nm light does not penetrate sufficiently at those depths to permit activation of the polymerization reaction) – the resulting restoration may then be described as having a 'soggy bottom'. Note, resin composites cure most efficiently closest to the 470 nm light source. Thus, angled incremental layering is a clinical technique deployed to minimize these negative effects.

6

6.2.3 The tooth–composite interface

Table 6.1 highlights some of the clinically important histological features of sound enamel and dentine relevant to the restoration of tooth surfaces with modern adhesive materials. An understanding of the interactions between the chemistry of the materials and this relevant histology is vital in order to optimize the qualities of the adhesive restorative systems available, including resin composites. Table 6.2 outlines the clinical properties that each layer of dental hard tissue confers to the crown of a tooth and those properties that a restorative material should exhibit to act as an ideal replacement material for each.

Table 6.1 Clinically relevant histology that might interact with the chemistry of modern adhesive restorative materials

	Mineral (inorganic)	Matrix (organic)	Structural arrangement
Enamel	Calcium hydroxyapatite crystallites ($Ca_{10}(PO_4)_6(OH)_2$ – $40 \times 60 \times 160$ nm) 96%weight, 89%vol.	No collagen. Enamelins (MW 55 kDa), amelogenins (MW 25 kDa) – 1%weight, 2%vol. Water – 3%weight, 9%vol.	10 000 crystallites arranged into *prisms* (US-rods); EDJ to surface; ameloblasts – Tomes' processes; 4–7 µm diameter; undulation, decussation; keyhole pattern in cross-section; prism cores/boundaries exist due to change in orientation of crystallites. Aprismatic layer at tooth surface on eruption.
Dentine	Calcium hydroxyapatite crystallites (with Mg and CO_3 substitutions – $5 \times 30 \times 80$ nm) β-octocalcium phosphate crystals.	90% collagen: Type I ($[\alpha_1(I)]_2\alpha_2(I)$) with trace amounts of type I trimer ($[\alpha_1(I)]_3$), 300 nm rod-shaped triple helical collagen molecules linearly aligned and cylindrically grouped as fibrils. Parallel fibrils gathered into fibres. 10% non-collagenous proteins (phosphorylated phosphoproteins (MW 140 kDa), Gla-proteins, macromolecular proteoglycans, plasma proteins, acidic glycoproteins), water.	*Tubules* (EDJ to pulp chamber); approx 19–45 000 per mm²; coronal sigmoid curvature; 1–5 µm diameter; anastomosing branches evident (0.5 µm – 25 nm diameter); odontoblasts and processes.

MW, molecular weight; kDa – kilo-Daltons; EDJ, enamel–dentine junction.

Table 6.2 Clinical properties that each of the dental hard tissues confers on a tooth and those properties an ideal restorative material should mimic

	Enamel	Enamel–dentine junction	Dentine
Clinical properties	Rigidity/brittle High compressive strength Wear resistance Translucency value Dry	Scalloped Optical tint Limits crack propagation/catastrophic failure 50 MPa bond strength	Bulk Slight elasticity/flexibility Shade Dynamic hydration – wetter, closer to the pulp (affect bonding ability)
Restorative replacement material	Dental composite	Dentine bonding agent Dynamic chemical bond	Glass ionomer cement

Resin composite and enamel

Hydrophobic resin composites adhere to dry enamel micro-mechanically and the prismatic, crystalline ultrastructure of enamel permits this to happen successfully, reliably and strongly (20–40 MPa bond strengths in laboratory studies). Three stages are required to develop the bond between composite and enamel after the enamel has been prepared mechanically during cavity preparation:

1. Acid etching (alternative US term – 'conditioning') – this is the process of placing 37% orthophosphoric acid gel onto the prepared enamel surface for 20 seconds. This:

– Removes surface contaminants (saliva, proteinaceous substances) and the smear layer (a tenacious surface layer of organic and inorganic cutting debris <50 μm thick) and increases surface area for bonding.

– Produces micro-irregularities/micro-porosities in the prismatic enamel surface. This microscopic surface roughness will provide micro-mechanical retention for the resin (see Figure 6.4).

2. After washing the acid-etch gel off and drying the enamel thoroughly, a layer of fluid unfilled hydrophobic bonding resin (that is, the resin without filler particles) is placed onto the etched enamel surface. This resin can flow easily into the micro-undercuts created by the etching process and it is then light cured. Note, the chemistry of the unfilled fluid bonding resin is not the same as that for a dentine bonding agent (see later).

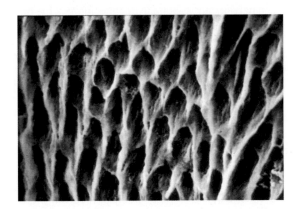

Figure 6.4 The tooth's view of an acid-etch retained bonding resin. The enamel was etched, washed, bonded, but then dissolved away in strong acids. The acid-resistant resin can be seen to have flowed into the prism boundary regions (field width 80 μm). (Courtesy of Professor A Boyde.)

3. The final composite can then be placed on the layer of cured bonding resin, in small angled increments (to lessen the effects of polymerization shrinkage) and cured to form the final contoured restoration (see Figure 6.5).

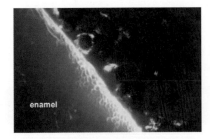

Figure 6.5 The interface between etched and bonded enamel prisms and a restoration. The bonding agent has been labelled with a yellow fluorescent dye (fluorescein) and its penetration around the horseshoe-shaped enamel prisms can be seen. Enamel prisms are easily separated from one another in the lateral walls of a cavity such as this, especially if the restoration shrinks (field width 500 μm).

When bonding to enamel at the margins of a cavity, consideration must be given to the quality of the prismatic structure. Prisms that have been sectioned/cracked/pulled apart during rotary instrumentation and whose bases do not reach the enamel–dentine junction (EDJ) intact are described as being *unsupported*. These prisms are inherently weak and if bonded to, will pull apart physically under the stresses exerted on them by the curing composite. This will lead to relatively short-term marginal failure within the enamel, i.e. cohesive enamel failure. In theory, if supported prisms are cut at, or close to, 90° to their long axis (i.e. clinically, the enamel margin is lightly bevelled), then the deleterious effects of shrinkage stress at the margins may be reduced as prisms possess greater tensile and compressive strengths along their c-axes, as opposed to perpendicular to the c-axes. Enamel that has lost much of the underlying dentine beneath it (*undermined* enamel) will need to have this replaced with a suitable material prior to the composite–enamel bond being created.

Resin composite and dentine: dentine bonding agents

The fundamental clinical problem is to achieve intimate compatibility of two immiscible substrates: dentine is hydrophilic (likes water and is innately wet), whereas methacrylate resins are hydrophobic (water-hating). Therefore, a *dentine bonding agent (DBA)* is required as an adhesive between the two. DBAs have three generic components:

● *Etch*: the first stage of the process, which has the following effects on dentine:

– Removes dentine smear layer created by the cavity preparation process (see Figure 6.6)

– Helps to unblock and widen the dentine tubule orifices

– Demineralizes the dentine surface so exposing the network of collagen in the dentine matrix (Table 6.1).

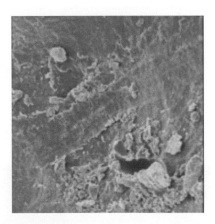

Figure 6.6 Dentine smear layer (a tenacious layer of organic and inorganic cutting debris usually 20 μm thick) imaged using scanning electron microscopy: this can be a barrier to good bonding and is normally removed/modified using acids (field width 500 μm).

Q6.6: How is the smear layer created?

- *Primer*: a bi-functional coupling molecule (e.g. hydrophilic HEMA – hydroxyethylmethacrylate), which has one functional group that is water-liking, so is compatible with the moist collagen in dentine, and another that is resin-liking, so is compatible with the bond/composite. The primer is carried into the moist collagen fibrillar network using a solvent (water, acetone, or alcohol), displacing the water molecules from the collagen and permitting the primer to enter into the micro- and nano-spaces created around the collagen fibrils after the etching process.

- *Bond*: this can be simply considered as the resin component of the composite without the filler particles. A soup of low viscosity monomers able to penetrate the spaces occupied by the primer monomers, it can be cured in the conventional way and then finally, the composite placed incrementally (chemically cross-linking to the monomers in the air-inhibited layer of the bond) and restoration completed.

Each of these sensitive stages needs to be accomplished in optimal clinical conditions to enable a successful bond to be created between composite and dentine. The status of the collagen network on the cut dentine surface is of prime importance – it is the penetration of the primer and bond into these micro-/nano-spaces that provide the integrity of the seal and bond between composite and dentine. This zone of collagen penetration is known as the *hybrid zone* and can be between 0.5 μm and 15 μm thick. Note, the thickness of the hybrid zone is less important than its continuity along the bonding interface. Any significant gaps in the hybrid zone will reduce the quality of the seal and ultimately the bond. Penetration of the bonding agent into the dentine tubules will also play a part in reinforcing the bond strength (see Figure 6.7). DBAs can also be used on enamel instead of the unfilled bonding resin described in the previous section, to simplify the overall bonding process, but note the chemistries of unfilled bonding resin (for enamel only) and DBAs (for both dentine and enamel) are different. There are numerous clinical presentations of DBAs from different manufacturers and a simple classification system dependent on the three stages described above is presented in Table 6.3. In Chapter 7, a further table is presented detailing the differences in the clinical techniques employed for each type of system (Table 7.12).

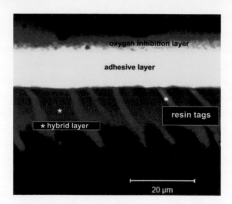

Figure 6.7 A fluorescent micrograph of a dentine bonding agent, showing penetration of the red-labelled (rhodamine) primer into the collagen network and tubules in dentine, forming the hybrid zone up to 15 μm thick (nano-retention) as well as resin tags (micro-retention). The yellow-labelled (fluorescein) adhesive uses its oxygen-inhibition layer to help adherence to the composite. (Courtesy of S Sauro.)

6.2.4 Types of dentine bonding agents – classification

Three-bottle or three-step bonding system   Where each of the three clinical stages is completed separately. Ideally, dentine should be etched for 10 seconds and enamel for 20 seconds using 37% orthophosphoric acid, which is then thoroughly washed (10 seconds) and dried until the enamel appears frosty white. The primer contains water so the over-dried exposed collagen on the dentine surface will rehydrate up to a point so permitting the primer and bond to penetrate the collagen network. However, over-etching coupled with incomplete rehydration of the collagen might leave unfilled micro-/nano-porosities within the depth of the hybrid zone and subsequent fluid movement might lead to postoperative sensitivity and bond degradation over time. Even though the clinical technique sensitivity is greater for type 1 systems due to the three separate steps, it is universally accepted that type 1, three-bottle systems provide a good quality and reliable bond

Table 6.3 A classification system for modern dentine bonding agents indicating the effect on the smear layer, presentation options of the three stages, etch, primer and bond, with some current UK market examples

Type	Smear layer	Etch	Primer	Bond	Clinical examples
1 (4th generation)	Remove				Scotchbond MP, Optibond FL
2 (5th generation)	Remove				Optibond Solo, Prime&Bond NT, XP Bond, iBond TE, Scotchbond 1-XT
3 (6th generation)	Dissolve	Weak self-etching primer			Liner Bond 2V, Clearfil SE, Silorane SE*
4 (7th generation)	Dissolve	Strong self-etching primer			Adper L-Pop Prompt, Xeno III, iBond, One Up Bond F Plus, G Bond

*This is an example of a strong self-etching primer used in a two-bottle system.

and have been used as the gold standard measurement in laboratory studies for dentine bonding.

Two-bottle or two-stage, 'total etch' or 'etch and rinse' adhesives The clinical stages have been simplified into two steps: an initial etch, as above, which is rinsed away so removing the smear layer. In type 2 systems it is imperative not to over-dry the exposed collagen network as this cannot be rehydrated by the contents of the second bottle containing both the primer and the bond (see Figure 6.8).

A technique of 'moist bonding' must be employed after washing the etchant gel off, wicking the 'puddles' of excess water away using cotton wool pledgets, paper points, or very gentle air drying (see Chapter 7). This will ensure the collagen network remains erect and supported, more conducive for bond penetration (see Figure 6.9). The primer and bond are combined and it is essential to evaporate the solvent carrier (acetone or alcohol) as any remnants will contaminate and weaken the final bond. This procedure also thins the adhesive on the cavity walls and the operator must ensure that there is enough adhesive present

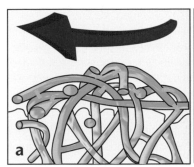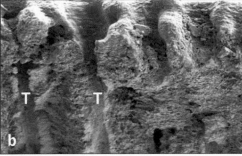

Figure 6.8 (**a**) Diagram showing collagen fibres in dentine that have been over-dried after etching. They have collapsed so neither the primer or bond can penetrate into the nano-spaces within the collagen network (red arrow). (Courtesy of D Ziskind.) (**b**) A scanning electron micrograph (field width 65 μm) showing an over-dried cut dentine surface with a collapsed collagen network (T, dentine tubule cut longitudinally). (**c**) Fluorescent confocal microscopic image (field width 250 μm) showing the bonding agent labelled with rhodamine (red). The resin composite can be seen in the top half of the image and the very faint outlines of dentinal tubules in the lower half. Note, as the dentine has been over-dried (see **a**), there has been no penetration of the collagen network or tubules and the resulting bond and seal will be poor.

Q6.8: What are the dark irregular shapes outlined within the rhodamine-labelled (red portion) of Figure 6.8?

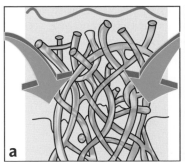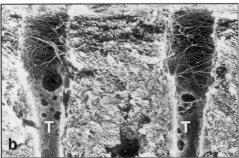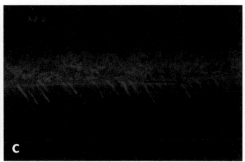

Figure 6.9 (**a**) Diagram showing collagen fibres in dentine that have been kept moist so the network is upright with micro-/nano-spaces available to accept the primer and bond (green arrows) (courtesy of D Ziskind). (**b**) An environmental scanning electron micrograph (field width 65 μm) showing moist collagen on the cut dentine surface. Individual collagen fibrils can be easily detected and the orifices of two tubules have been clearly widened by the etching process (T, dentine tubule cut longitudinally) (courtesy of Bart van Meerbeek). (**c**) Fluorescent confocal microscopic image (field width 250 μm) showing the bonding agent labelled with a red dye penetrating the moist collagen network on the dentine surface (nano-mechanical retention) and into the tubules (micro-mechanical retention). Note the thin red diffuse band at the interface between dentine and composite (arrow), this is the *hybrid zone* (10 μm thick).

before the curing stage (the cavity walls will appear shiny). Therefore, multiple applications of the adhesive (primer and bond together) may be required prior to placing the composite restoration.

Weaker self-etching primers The acidic phosphate monomers in the primer act as the etchant so no separate etch/rinsing/drying phase or moist bonding technique is required. The dentine is etched sufficiently to dissolve partially the smear layer and expose the collagen network. The enamel margins may be etched less efficiently, however, thus leading to a distinct possibility of stained margins of restorations in the long term (see Figure 6.10).

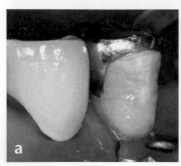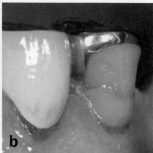

Figure 6.10 (**a**) Resin composite class V buccal cervical restoration LL5 placed using a type 3 self-etching primer dentine bonding agent. (**b**) The same restoration, 10 years later.

> **Q6.10:** Can you spot the difference between the two restorations and explain the reason for the difference?

This problem may be prevented by pre-etching the enamel margins with 37% orthophosphoric acid for 15 seconds, converting the whole clinical process similar to a type 1, three-stage system (Chapter 7). The solvent again must be evaporated after the acidic primer is rubbed onto the dentine surface as in the type 2 systems. An exception to the weak self-etching type 3 systems is the silorane bonding system from 3MESPE. This contains a strong self-etching, relatively hydrophilic primer, which needs to be light cured before the separate, very hydrophobic bond is applied. This bonding agent is marketed for the sole purpose of bonding a low-shrink composite, Filtek Silorane (see Section 6.2.6).

Stronger self-etching all-in-one systems Clinically, the simplest to use as there is a single application step but the three bonding stages (etch, prime, and bond) are somewhat compromised. These are the latest systems on the market and currently there are no long-term data. Laboratory studies on sound enamel and dentine show not only favourable bond strengths but also the presence of water blisters in the adhesive layer as the bond acts as a semi-permeable membrane, drawing water from the wet dentine tubules. As hydrolysis of polymeric dentine bonds is a known problem, it will be interesting to see how these findings relate to longer-term clinical outcomes.

6.2.5 Issues with dentine bonding agents

- *Technique sensitivity*: the steps involved in dentine bonding require high levels of moisture control intraorally and appropriate handling of the dental materials themselves. For example, if volatile solvents are allowed to evaporate naturally from bottles of adhesive when lids are not replaced after dispensing, the chemistry is irreversibly adversely affected so bonding will be impaired. Primers and bond need to be agitated well into the tooth surface and all these steps must be followed to obtain a successful bond.

- *Packaging instructions*: familiarization with the steps in the bonding process is essential and teamwork with the nurse is vital in order to place the various materials in the correct order, with speed and precision. Single dose capsules/foils/bubble-packs can be of assistance, reducing wastage and improving infection control procedures.

- *Shelf-life*: if kept refrigerated, the shelf-life of most DBAs is good. Volatile solvents need to be kept tightly stoppered, and as materials are light sensitive, blacked-out bottles are advised.

- *Suitable substrate*: most studies on DBAs use sound enamel and dentine as the tooth surface to which to bond, often on extracted teeth. The histological properties of teeth *in vivo* may be quite different and also the quality of the hard tissues will vary depending on the amount of carious tooth structure that has been retained. Therefore, a comprehensive understanding is required of the state of the collagen network and mineral prior to using the DBA. More recent publications have used caries-affected dentine substrates *in vitro* and show acceptable bond strengths (15–28 MPa).

- *Hydrolysis*: The major factor in the long-term degradation of the bond interface. The residual monomers will be affected by the water transition through vital dentine, so ultimately compromising the seal and bond. Therefore, a good quality peripheral enamel seal is essential for the long-term success of adhesive bonding. Matrix metalloproteinases (MMPs) released from the exposed collagen (Chapter 1), and activated in the acidic environment, may account for the failure of the adhesive bond in both caries-affected and sound dentine.

- *Sensitization*: These chemicals are designed to penetrate living tissue and latex or nitrile gloves do not offer protection from resin-based materials. Therefore, the dentist and nurse need to follow a 'no-touch' regimen when handling these materials.

6.2.6 Developments

The world of dental materials is constantly changing and by the time this book is published new materials will be available to be used clinically. Some of the latest innovations/developments are discussed below.

Low-shrink composites

Manufacturers are attempting to alleviate the problem of significant volumetric shrinkage (often leading to increased marginal stress and/or material strain). 3MESPE has produced Filtek Silorane posterior composite; a packable, posterior composite based primarily upon siloxane-oxirane (silorane) chemistry, as opposed to conventional methacrylates. In this system, the monomers, instead of being linear, are ring-opening so, during the cationic polymerization process, less shrinkage occurs (0.9%). This chemistry requires a separate bonding agent, Filtek Silorane Bond, which is very hydrophobic, so minimizing the water transition through the adhesive. Septodont has developed a dimer-acid nano-hybrid composite (based on dimer dicarbamate dimethacrylates), which exhibits phase separation (expansion) on curing so reducing some of the effects of polymerization shrinkage.

Dentine bonding agents

With the advent of low-shrink composites, the importance of direct bond strengths may lessen and more emphasis would be placed on the ionic interaction between the materials and tooth structure. Medicinal ions could be transferred from the adhesive to help remineralize the enamel or dentine or act as antibacterial agents.

'Self-adhesive composite'

The ultimate development, a simple to use, self-adhesive reliable restorative material that could help regenerate the hard tooth tissues.

6.3 Glass ionomer cement

Glass ionomer cement (GIC) is a water-based, plastic direct dental restorative cement formed from an acid–base reaction between a poly-alkenoic acid and ion-leachable fluoro-calcium (strontium) aluminosilicate glass particles.

6.3.1 History

GIC was developed as a biocompatible, chemically adhesive plastic restorative material by Wilson and Kent in the UK in 1972.

6.3.2 Chemistry

- *Powder*: calcium fluoro-aluminosilicate glass particles with strontium (to increase radio-opacity). The silica (SiO_2 – affecting transparency), alumina (Al_2O_3 – affecting opacity, setting time, and can increase the compressive strength of the set cement) and calcium fluoride (CaF_2 – the fluoride ions reduce the fusion temperature, increase strength of the set cement, enhance translucency, and have a therapeutic effect) are the important components. These are structured ionically as a tetrahedron complex with a centrally located aluminium ion and closely localized alkaline earth cations (sodium, potassium, calcium, and strontium) to maintain electro-neutrality.

- *Liquid-polyacid*: itaconic acid copolymer solution in water plus tartaric acid (5–15%, maintains working time and assists setting reaction). Anhydrous forms have vacuum-dried polyacrylic acid incorporated into the powder and are mixed with water ± dilute solution of tartaric acid.

- *Setting reaction*: acid–base reaction with three stages:

1. *Dissolution*: sol formation from the outer layers of the glass particles as they are attacked by the polyacid and calcium, strontium, aluminium, and fluoride ions are released.

2. *Gelation and hardening*: primarily calcium ions bind to carboxylate groups (4–5 minutes) producing a clinically hard surface (initial set) and a silaceous hydrogel is formed, maturing over 24 hours, with further cross-linking with aluminium ions, up to 7 days. This process causes volumetric shrinkage of up to 3%. Surface protection at this stage is advisable to ensure regulation of water molecules in and out of the hydrogel, so permitting maturation to occur.

3. *Hydration*: associated with phase 2, this continues over 4–6 months, so improving the physical properties of the material. The uptake of water leads to a balancing expansion, so reducing the ill effects of the initial shrinkage.

6.3.3 The tooth–GIC interface

GICs have the ability to adhere chemically to mineralized dental tissues. They do this by the dynamic processes of diffusion and adsorption.

Enamel GIC polyacid displaces phosphate and divalent Ca ions from the hydroxyapatite and these ions become incorporated into the GIC matrix, which sets, pH rises and re-precipitation of minerals at the GIC/tooth interface occurs, forming an ion-enriched layer, so firmly bound that when GIC restorations fail, this can be cohesive within the GIC material itself (see Figure 6.11). If the enamel prisms have been damaged/fractured/pulled apart in creating the cavity, the mineralized component of the interface can also fail cohesively due to the initial shrinkage stresses generated by the setting GIC (see Figure 6.12).

Dentine–collagen Adhesion to collagen may occur through hydrogen bond formation or metallic ion bridging between carboxyl groups of the polyacid and collagen molecules.

Dentine–tubules There is limited evidence to argue for any significant micro-mechanical retention by the penetration of dentine tubules. The penetration is slight (<5 μm) and the tensile strength of GIC in this proportion is poor, so unlikely to contribute towards retention.

6

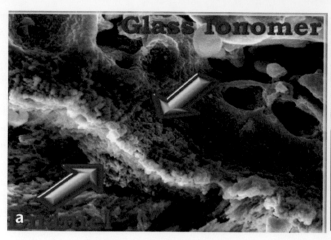
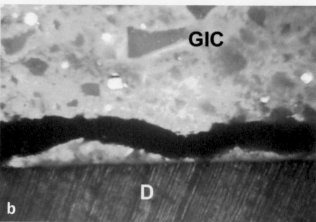

Figure 6.11 (a) Scanning electron microscopy image showing interface between glass ionomer and enamel. The section surface has been lightly etched and a raised area (between the arrows) shows the *ion-enriched* layer at the tooth/restoration interface (field width 10 μm). (Courtesy of Dr Hien Ngo.) (b) Fractured GIC/tooth interface (D) showing the cohesive failure common to these materials. The *ion-enriched* layer is still attached to the tooth (field width 300 μm).

Q6.11: What is responsible for the cohesive fracture in Figure 6.11b?

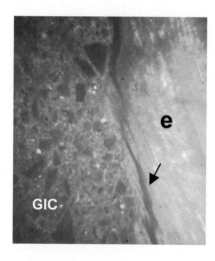

Figure 6.12 Photomicrograph of glass ionomer cement having pulled apart enamel prisms and caused cohesive failure in the enamel (e; black arrow) (field width 100 μm).

Q6.12: What are the irregular-shaped particles within the GIC?

Conditioning

Conditioning is the process by which both enamel and dentine are 'freshened' or preactivated prior to the placement of freshly mixed GIC. The acid used is 10% polyacrylic acid for 10 seconds, which is then washed off and the surface lightly dried, to:

- Remove/modify the smear layer and expose calcium and phosphate ions on the mineralized surface.

- Reduce the surface energy of the tooth surface to allow improved wettability of the GIC as it is placed on the tooth surface.

It is mildly acidic, so neither demineralizes the dentine excessively, nor opens up dentine tubules. Note, this conditioning step is not the same as the 'conditioners' used in resin composite retention – that material, even though sharing the same nomenclature, is a much stronger acid etch (37% orthophosphoric acid).

6.3.4 Clinical uses of GIC relating to its properties

GICs are conventionally used as:

- Luting cements for indirect restorations, where the powder to liquid ratio is closer to 1.5:1 (less viscosity to improve cavity margin adaptation).

- Direct restorative material, with a powder:liquid ratio >3:1 (stiffer material).

- Indirect pulp protection – powder:liquid ratio, 1.5:1, covering a direct pulp capping agent (e.g. calcium hydroxide or MTA) or in the depths of a cavity with very close proximity to the pulp (see Chapter 5).

As a restorative material, the best physical properties (tensile and compressive strengths) of GIC are exhibited when the material is used in thicker sections, but GICs are still not universally recommended for long-term stress-bearing restorations (e.g. posterior occlusal restorations). Internal cavity line angles should be smooth and rounded prior to placement.

- *Fracture resistance*: original GICs were brittle and prone to fracture under heavy occlusal loading. Modern derivatives have an improved fracture toughness but there is still little clinical evidence and justification for them being used routinely as long-term restorations in the posterior load-bearing dentition.

- *Abrasion resistance*: again, generally poor but modern resin-based coating systems can help regulate the long-term water uptake and provide a protective and aesthetic coating so improving this quality.

- *Physical properties*: compressive, shear strengths, thermal expansion and diffusivity have all improved with developments in GIC science and modern materials appear to have properties approaching more closely those of natural dentine.

- *Fluoride release*: fluoride ions are released initially at high levels, which fall away 8–10 weeks after placement. The fluoride ions are captured within the siliceous hydrogel matrix and can pass in and out of this to the tooth surface, so prompting the description that it can act as a 'fluoride reservoir', recharging from the high doses of professional fluoride application. There is contrary evidence that argues the fluoride release effect is subclinical after initial placement.

- *Aesthetics*: improvements have been made with better shade and translucency of modern GICs. Water uptake and high solubility affect the long-term stability of colour and translucency in restorations but coating the surface just after placement or veneering the surface with composite at a later date, are potential solutions.

6.3.5 Developments

As with dental composites, GIC material science is continuously evolving. Developments are being made:

- In the speed, control and conversion rate of the initial set, with fast-setting materials on the market taking 90 seconds to reach a carvable stage.

- Improving the physical properties in order to enable reliable use in posterior, load-bearing cavities with the potential use of ceramic nano-filler technology or developing the use of N-vinyl pyrollidone-containing polyacids (NVPs) in the matrix polymer.

- Improving the wear resistance, polishability, and aesthetics of the final restoration with advances in resin-based coating systems, applied after finishing the restoration.

- Greater use of the ionic exchange potential to introduce other ions to help remineralize, repair tooth structure, and confer antibacterial effects.

6.4 Resin-modified glass ionomer cement (RM-GIC) and polyacid modified resin composite ('compomer')

The description of these materials as 'light-cured GICs' should be avoided.

6.4.1 Chemistry

RM-GICs

RM-GICs essentially contain the same chemistry as a conventional GIC with the addition of the hydrophilic resin, HEMA (hydroxyethylmethacrylate), bis-GMA, and other photo-initiators. They set with a combination reaction: acid–base between the glass particles and polyalkenoic acid (as previously described) and also light-cured polymerization reaction of the resin (similar to that of a resin composite). The resin in RM-GICs can also undergo chemical polymerization due to an intrinsic redox (reduction-oxidation) reaction so will auto-cure over time (approximately 1 month) into a fully set material. Due to the fact that the HEMA resin is hydrophilic, there is a risk that after the initial snap-setting process, water is absorbed which might lead to medium- to long-term degradation and colour instability when used as the definitive restorative material. Clinical examples include Fuji II LC, Vitremer, and Ketac Nano.

Polyacid modified composites

These are materials that are primarily resin based, with some GIC chemistry but not enough to promote an acid–base setting reaction. These materials essentially require light activation to promote the polymerization chain reaction. They cannot chemically adhere to tooth structure as do conventional GICs, as the acid–base reaction only occurs over a prolonged time, after the initial set of the resin component. Therefore dentine bonding agents are a pre-requisite for retention of these materials within a cavity. Clinical examples include Dyract and Compoglass.

6.4.2 Clinical indications

Both of these materials can be used as provisional or definitive shade-matched tooth-coloured adhesive restoratives. However, there is some evidence that the colour stability of RM-GICs might be suspect over longer periods due to the water absorption that occurs (see Figure 6.13).

RM-GICs may also be used as a base in an adhesive *layered/laminate/*'*sandwich*' restoration with an overlying composite completely covering the RM-GIC base (a closed restoration). However, there is clinical evidence that these types of restoration are more prone

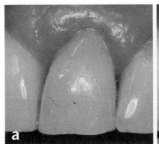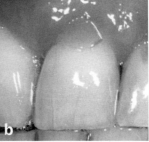

Figure 6.13 (a) RM-GIC buccal cervical Class V restoration UL1 with good aesthetic properties initially. **(b)** Same restoration 6 years later showing obvious intrinsic discoloration due to water absorption.

to long-term failure especially at the interfaces between differing materials. It is of the authors' opinion that the *layered/laminate/sandwich* restoration should be limited to the placement of a composite veneer over the exposed, occlusal surface of large GICs/RM-GICs at least 6 months after the GIC restoration has been placed to allow for its full maturation, so maximizing its physical and chemical properties.

6.5 Dental amalgam

Dental amalgam (one of the oldest direct restorative materials still in use) is an alloy of one or more metals including silver (Ag), tin (Sn), zinc (Zn), copper (Cu), and tiny amounts of some minor elements (palladium, platinum, indium) with mercury (Hg). Its use is rapidly on the decline worldwide as:

- Patients demand more aesthetic restorations and can appreciate the benefits of simple restore/repair cycles of treatment.
- Health and safety and environmental issues are raised against the use and disposal of mercury.
- Adhesive materials have developed with significantly improved bonding abilities to sound and carious tooth structure.
- Principles of minimally invasive dentistry have been embraced, producing smaller, less mechanically retentive cavities to restore, so promoting the use of adhesive materials.
- Caries control/management strategies have evolved with a better understanding of the histopathology of the disease.

6.5.1 Chemistry

- Silver (65–70%), tin (26–29%), copper (<6% low Cu, >12% high Cu) and trace metallic elements (<1%) are presented as phases: γ gamma (Ag_3Sn), ε epsilon (Cu_3Sn) and d dispersant (Ag-Cu eutectic alloy) and mixed with mercury (triturated in an amalgamator unit) to form an alloy (amalgamation reaction) so producing the intrinsic strength and mechanical properties of the set material.
- Metal phases are presented as ingots which are then made into lathe-cut particles. Alternatively, molten alloy is sprayed into an inert atmosphere and atomized into spherical particles. The final powder may be an admix of the two particle types. The particle size and shape has an effect on the ease of packing the triturated amalgam into a cavity; spherical particle alloys require less force to condense into a cavity resulting in fewer voids.
- Copper: modern alloys are high Cu alloys with >12% Cu (single composition or dispersion-modified Cu enriched alloys). It improves corrosion and creep resistance and strengthens the set material by reducing unwanted Sn-Hg γ_2 (gamma 2) phase in the set amalgam.
- Zinc: >0.01% was introduced to scavenge oxygen when casting the metal ingots. Use of an inert atmosphere now makes the inclusion of zinc redundant. Inclusion of zinc led to increased hygroscopic expansion due to water contamination during placement but may increase marginal strength.

6.5.2 Physical properties

- *Strength*: high compressive and tensile strengths several days after placement. Care is required when checking the occlusion immediately after condensation and carving as the amalgam may be brittle at this stage. High Cu alloys have a greater strength and are used in large load-bearing posterior restorations. Amalgam is weak in thin section and requires at least 2 mm thickness to support itself. Therefore cavity design is important for this reason as well as for mechanical retention via undercuts.
- *Corrosion*: an electrochemical breakdown due to the interaction between any metal and its surroundings. Low Cu amalgams corroded quickly and extensively so sealing the gap between the cavity wall and restoration. High Cu alloys are more resistant to corrosion and corrosion fatigue at the margins. Amalgam surfaces can oxidize over time leading to surface corrosion or even breakdown leading to pitting and surface deficiencies.
- *Rigidity*: the modulus of elasticity of amalgam is high but not as rigid as enamel.
- *Dimensional changes*: after minor setting contraction, water uptake during setting (especially in low Cu, Zn-containing alloys) can lead to hydrogen production and expansion leading to pain. Thermal expansion can also occur to a degree further than normal tooth structure so fine surface polishing, the friction of which will generate heat, should be undertaken with due care.

6.5.3 Bonded and sealed amalgams

Amalgam restorations obtain retention within a cavity macro-mechanically, achieved by making undercut preparations (where the base of the cavity is wider than its opening) or using slots/grooves, root canal posts or the pulp chamber and root canal orifices themselves (Nayyar core, Figure 6.14). All of these require excessive tooth structure to be removed or damaged to some extent, so ultimately weakening the remaining tissue. Dentine pins have been used to retain amalgam in larger cavities where cusps are missing. There is clear evidence that correct placement of dentine pins tends to increase significantly the stresses in an already weakened tooth, leading to catastrophic failure of the restoration and tooth. It is the authors' opinion that dentine pins should not be used in modern dentistry as alternative methods and materials now exist, including self-curing adhesive luting cements to couple the cavity walls with the amalgam.

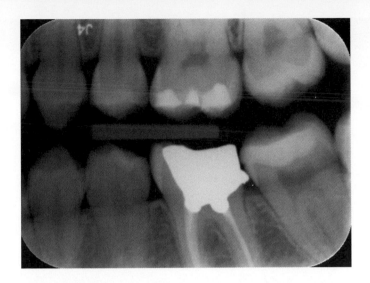

Figure 6.14 Left bitewing radiograph showing an amalgam Nayyar core LL6. Note how the 'amalgam pins' extend into the coronal aspects of the endodontically treated root canals, to aid retention after the gutta percha was removed. The bulk of amalgam will also confer strength to the restoration. For the clinical steps to place a Nayyar core, see Chapter 7.

> **Q6.14:** What problem can you see with this restoration and how can it be treated? What do you think should be considered as part of the long-term management of this tooth?

Bonded amalgams

An adhesive, chemically cured resin-based luting cement is used to seal the dentine tubules, bond to the dentine collagen (as with composites) and simultaneously micro-mechanically interlock with the freshly condensed amalgam as they both set. Chemical bonds with metal oxides forming in the set amalgam may form, but these have little clinical significance for retention in the long term. The evidence for their routine use is inconclusive, but the procedure might be beneficial when repairing old fractured large amalgams with new amalgam.

Sealed amalgams

As modern high Cu alloys corrode less and so do not adequately seal the spaces at the tooth–amalgam interface, a flowable resin/dentine bonding agent can be used to coat the surface of the tooth–amalgam interface after condensation, carving, and finishing. This can penetrate the micro-gaps at the marginal interface which form during the setting process, so reducing the chance of marginal leakage and the risk of subsequent caries. A dentine bonding agent may also be used to seal the dentine cavity walls prior to placement of the amalgam restoration.

6.5.4 Modern indications for the use of amalgam

In the current climate of more acceptable tooth-coloured alternatives and minimally invasive dentistry as well as the ever stronger push towards the environmental concerns over the safety and disposal of mercury, the use of dental amalgam is becoming more limited. Due to the presence of alternatives, the use of amalgam may reasonably be restricted to large posterior load-bearing restorations or as a core material for crowns (Chapter 7).

6

6.6 Temporary (intermediate) and provisional restorative materials

6.6.1 Characteristics

Temporary restorative materials should ideally be:

- Simple for both the dentist and nurse to handle clinically
- Easy to remove to allow final placement of the definitive restoration
- Materials that do not interfere with the setting/bonding chemistry of any definitive restorative material
- Durable enough to last in the oral cavity for several weeks
- Cheap, biocompatible.

  Provisional restorative materials should ideally be all of the above and:

- Durable enough to last in the oral cavity for several months
- As aesthetic as possible.

  The boundary between a provisional and definitive restorative material is nowadays quite blurred as many adhesive materials combine both functions.

6.6.2 Chemistry

- Radio-opaque, polymer-reinforced zinc oxide: eugenol cements (e.g. Kalzinol, Sedanol, pre-mixed Intermediate Restorative Material – IRM). Quick setting and easy to spatulate and load into cavities, but must not be used where resin composites will follow as the eugenol affects the polymerization chain reaction.
- Glass ionomer cements (see previous sections).
- Zinc polycarboxylate cements (Poly F Plus): water-soluble low-molecular-weight polymers of acrylic or methacrylic acid that form solid, insoluble products when mixed with specially prepared ZnO powder. The resulting cement adheres to dental enamel and can be also used as a luting agent.

6.7 Answers to self-test questions

Q6.1: What properties of the dental composite does monomer chain length affect?

A: The viscosity of the uncured material and the degree of polymerization shrinkage (see text).

Q6.6: How is the smear layer created?

A: By the friction generated from any cutting instrument on the tooth surface (hand instrument or rotary); air-abrasion produces a layer similar to a smear layer created from organic/inorganic chip debris and abrasive particles.

Q6.8: What are the dark irregular shapes outlined within the rhodamine-labelled (red portion) of the above image?

A: These are the irregular silica-based filler particles within the resin composite.

Q6.10: Can you spot the difference between the two restorations and explain the reason for the difference?

A: Note the dark discoloration on the superior margin of the restoration–enamel interface. This is due to the enamel not being as efficiently etched by the weaker self-etching primer. This has led to a less well sealed adhesive bond which has gradually picked up stain over the last decade of use. Pre-etching the enamel with 37% orthophosphoric acid etch can alleviate this problem.

Q6.11: What is responsible for the cohesive fracture in Figure 6.11b?

A: Phase 2 of the setting reaction with the formation of calcium and aluminium cross-links coupled with potential dehydration of the GIC.

Q6.12: What are the irregular-shaped particles within the GIC?

A: Unreacted fluoro-calcium aluminosilicate glass particles.

Q6.14: What problem can you see with this restoration and how can it be treated? What do you think should be considered as part of the long-term management of this tooth?

A: Note the distal amalgam overhang, caused by inadequate adaptation of the matrix band when originally packing the cavity. This may be removed using fine burs (if clinical access is available) and interproximal amalgam finishing strips. If not, the long-term management of the tooth may involve the placement of an indirect full coverage cast restoration (e.g. a metal ceramic or full gold crown) and during the tooth preparation for this, the overhang will be automatically removed.

6

7

Clinical operative procedures – a step-by-step guide

Chapter contents

7.1 Introduction

This chapter illustrates several operative dentistry procedures used for the successful placement of direct plastic restorations into the posterior and anterior dentition. The procedure list cannot be and is not exhaustive, but has been chosen to give the reader the broadest application of the techniques described. The techniques shown are not exclusive – there are many varied operative techniques to remove caries and place suitable restorations (Chapter 5), but the authors feel that the methods described are simple and achievable for most clinical abilities and in most clinical situations. The experienced skilled clinician is able to adapt the myriad of skills outlined in these examples to best fit the unfolding clinical situation presented to them.

7.1.1 Cavity/restoration classification

There are several classifications of cavities in the dental literature attempting to correlate site, size of lesion, and disease activity. The oldest, simplest, and probably most universal in acceptance is Black's classification (Table 7.1). This classification was originally used to denote the most common sites for caries to develop so helping to formulate an idea of the individual's caries risk. Nowadays, it is used to describe the site of the cavity or restoration and is useful for descriptive purposes, communicating between dentists or annotations in dental records. It must be understood that cavities should not be cut with predetermined geometric shapes according to this classification, but the classification should be used according to the final restoration placed, which will be governed by the biological extent of the caries, the type of material used, and other factors (e.g. amount/strength of tooth structure retained and occlusal factors).

Table 7.1 Black's classification of caries lesions – now often misused by dentists as a purely descriptive analysis of restoration site*

Black's class	Site
I	Posterior restoration contained within the occlusal surface
II	Posterior restoration including an approximal surface
III	Anterior restoration including an approximal surface only
IV	Anterior incisal edge restoration
V	Buccal cervical surface restoration

*Note that with the increased use of adhesive restoratives, many restorations may involve several of the listed sites and therefore need more specific, accurate descriptions.

7.1.2 Restoration procedures

The remainder of this chapter will be dedicated to describing and illustrating the practical stages in placing certain types of restoration, outlining in detail the clinical procedures involved (Tables 7.2–7.11). Discussion of the separate steps will be found throughout the preceding chapters and these links are given throughout. It is assumed that the clinical need for intervention has been appropriately ascertained and any necessary local analgesia has been administered prior to commencement of the restorative procedures outlined. (Note: abbreviations used in Tables 7.2–7.11 – CS, carbon steel; DBA, dentine bonding agent; GIC, glass ionomer cement; LCPA, long cone periapical radiograph; min, minutes; PA, periapical; RM, resin-modified; s, seconds; TC, tungsten carbide.)

7

7.2 Fissure sealant

Table 7.2 Operative procedure: fissure sealant

	Indication (Chapters 2,3)	Preoperative procedures/ isolation (Chapter 5)	Caries removal/ cavity preparation (Chapter 5)	Cavity modification (Chapter 5)	Bonding steps (Chapter 6)	Restorative steps	Finishing steps
Fissure sealant (FS) composite *GIC/RM-GIC*	High caries risk, deep fissure patterns, stagnating plaque. Newly erupting molars.	Rubber dam. (Cotton wool rolls/aspiration.)	Fissure debridement with prophypaste and rotating brush. Sodium bicarbonate air-polishing. Bioactive glass air-abrasion.	Wash and dry using 3-1 syringe (10 s).	*Composite:* 37% orthophosphoric acid etch enamel fissures (20 s), wash and dry (10 s). *GIC/RM-GIC:* 10% polyacrylic acid conditioning of enamel fissures (15 s), wash and dry (10 s).	*Composite:* FS flowed into fissure pattern, light cure (470 nm) for 20 s. *GIC/RM-GIC:* applied into fissure pattern, auto-cured/light cured (470 nm, 20 s).	Remove isolation. Check margins with probe. Check occlusion with articulating paper.

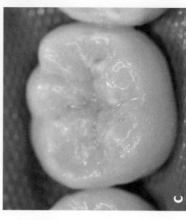

Figure 7.2 (a) Preoperative image of the occlusal surface of LR6 with deep fissures in a high caries risk individual.

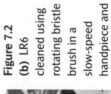

Figure 7.2 (b) LR6 cleaned using rotating bristle brush in a slow-speed handpiece and prophypaste.

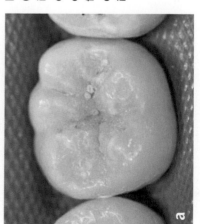

Figure 7.2 (c) LR6 post-cleaning.

Figure 7.2

(d) 37% orthophosphoric acid etch gel rubbed onto the enamel occlusal surface of the LR6 for 20 seconds.

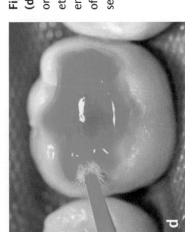

Figure 7.2

(f) Resin composite fissure sealant applied into fissures using a ball-ended dental probe. The sealant flows easily into the fissure pattern.

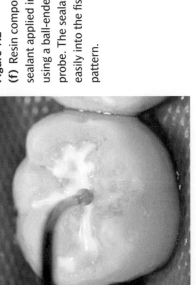

Figure 7.2

(h) Completed occlusal fissure sealant on the LR6.

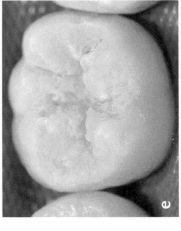

Figure 7.2

(e) Etch gel washed off for 10 seconds and air-dried using the 3-1 air/water syringe. Note the frosty appearance of etched occlusal enamel, indicating creation of micro-porosities which aid the micro-mechanical retention of the resin composite fissure sealant.

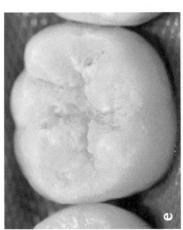

Figure 7.2

(g) Resin composite fissure sealant is light cured (470 nm wavelength light for 20 seconds) to initiate the addition polymerization reaction of the resin monomers.

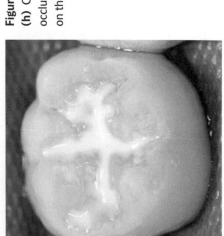

7

7.3 Preventive resin restoration (PRR), type 3 DBA (enamel pre-etch, see Chapter 6)

Table 7.3 Operative procedure: preventive resin restoration

	Indication (Chapters 2,3)	Preoperative procedures/ isolation (Chapter 5)	Caries removal/ cavity preparation (Chapter 5)	Cavity modification (Chapter 5)	Bonding steps (Chapter 6)	Restorative steps	Finishing steps
Preventive resin restoration (PRR) *Composite*	Same as for FS but evidence of enamel demineralization (mICDAS 1, 2).	Rubber dam. (Cotton wool rolls/ aspiration.)	Enamel fissure lesion excavated with 330 TC bur, air-turbine. (Air-abrasion – bioactive glass, alumina.)	Wash and dry using 3-1 syringe (10 s).	*Composite:* 37% orthophosphoric acid etch enamel fissures (20 s), wash and dry (10 s).	*Composite:* resin flowed into widened fissure, light cure (470 nm) for 20 s.	Remove isolation. Check margins with probe. Check occlusion with articulating paper.
GIC			Debride remaining fissures with prophy-paste/ rotating brush.		*GIC:* 10% polyacrylic acid conditioning of enamel fissures (15 s), wash and dry (10 s).	*GIC:* applied into widened fissure, auto-cure/light cured (470 nm, 20 s).	

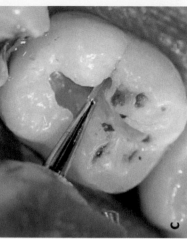

Figure 7.3 (a) Isolated LR7 with deep stained fissures, cavitated and carious in places in a high caries risk individual (mICDAS 3).

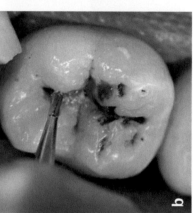

Figure 7.3 (b) Occlusal fissures explored with 330 bur in an air-turbine handpiece.

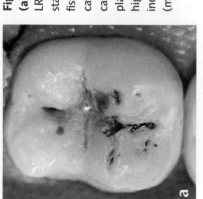

Figure 7.3 (c) Fissures widened and caries-infected dentine removed distally (soft, sticky). The mesial extent of the fissures opened within enamel.

Figure 7.3
(f) LR7 occlusal enamel pre-etched using 37% orthophosphoric acid etch gel for 15 s.

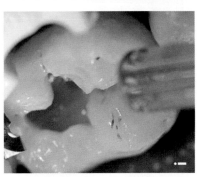

Figure 7.3
(i) Air-dried for 5–10 s to evaporate solvent (and thin the layer) until there is no visible 'rippling' of primer on tooth surface.

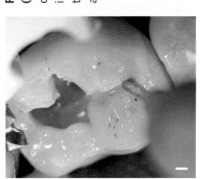

Figure 7.3
(l) Flowable resin composite directly introduced into the mesial fissure and light cured.

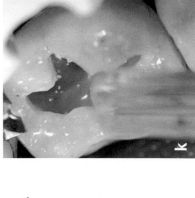

Figure 7.3
(e) Fine diamond bur is used to remove grossly unsupported enamel and lightly bevel the margins.

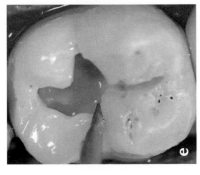

Figure 7.3
(h) Type 3 DBA applied (two-step, self-etching primer). Self-etching primer rubbed into all cavity surfaces for 10 s.

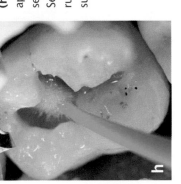

Figure 7.3
(k) Type 3 DBA bond/adhesive air-thinned as above. Note shiny cavity floor surface which should be seen before light curing (470 nm, 20 s).

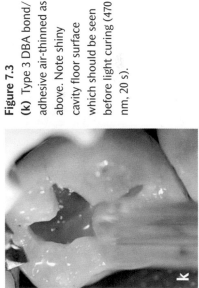

7

Figure 7.3
(d) Fissure pattern fully opened distally with caries-affected dentine retained at the cavity floor (scratchy but flaky).

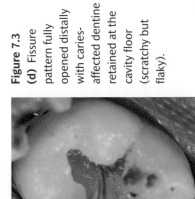

Figure 7.3
(g) Gel washed off for 10 s and gently air-dried (2–3 s).

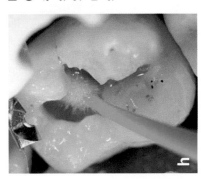

Figure 7.3
(j) Type 3 DBA bond/adhesive rubbed onto cavity surfaces.

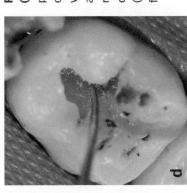

7

Figure 7.3

(n) Adapted using a burnisher (<2 mm increment), leaving space for next enamel shade increment. This is light cured, leaving uncured air-inhibited layer on composite surface ready to accept next increment.

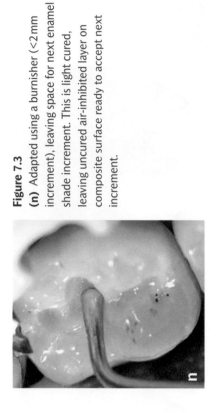

Figure 7.3

(p) Shaped and contoured using Ward's carver/a pear-shaped burnisher and subsequently light cured.

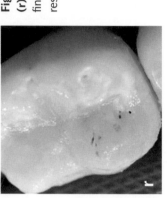

Figure 7.3

(r) The final finished PRR restoration LR7.

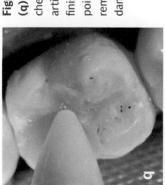

Figure 7.3

(m) Dentine shade resin composite introduced into distal cavity from compule.

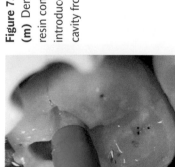

Figure 7.3

(o) Enamel shade resin composite directly introduced into the cavity.

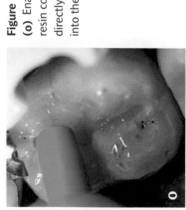

Figure 7.3

(q) The occlusion is checked using articulating paper and finished using polishing points and cups (after removing the rubber dam).

7.4 Posterior occlusal composite restoration (Class I), low-shrink silorane composite

Table 7.4 Operative procedure: posterior occlusal composite restoration (Class I)

Operative procedure 7.4	Indication (Chapters 2,3)	Preoperative procedures/isolation (Chapter 5)	Caries removal/cavity preparation (Chapter 5)	Cavity modification (Chapter 5)	Bonding steps (Chapter 6)	Restorative steps	Finishing steps
Posterior occlusal adhesive restoration: (Class I) All GIC All composite Old posterior occlusal GIC to be veneered with composite	High caries risk patient (mICDAS 2); cavitated lesion (mICDAS 3,4). Consider pulp response to sensibility tests. Radiographic assessment of pulp proximity. Assess occlusal integrity/wear/marginal failure of >6 month old posterior GIC restoration.	Check occlusion with articulating paper, preoperatively. Select tooth – material shade (Vita guides). Place rubber dam.	Remove central unsupported/undermined demineralized enamel with TC/diamond bur, air-turbine. Leave sound enamel margin. Peripheral dentine caries excavation (CS, slow-speed rose-head bur, hand excavator) to affected/sound dentine (lesion depth-dependent). Excavate infected dentine overlying pulp with hand excavator/avoid exposure. Remove 2 mm thickness of old, occlusal GIC with diamond/TC bur, air-turbine. Leave sound enamel margins.	Lightly bevel sound enamel margins using fine diamond bur, air-turbine. Gently round off internal cavity line angles using slow-speed CS rose-head burs. Wash and dry cavity (10 s).	*GIC:* 10% polyacrylic acid conditioner rubbed onto cavity walls with micro-brush (15 s), wash and dry (10 s) – removes smear layer and exposes Ca^{2+} ions for bonding. *Composite:* dependent on which DBA (types 1–4) used (Table 7.12).	Mix/dispense *GIC* into cavity, filling from base upwards (to prevent voids/improve adaptation to cavity walls). Slightly overfill cavity initially. After 60 s pack GIC into the cavity with burnisher/flat plastics ensuring adequate condensation. Occlusal morphology adapted with flat plastics and excess material removed while GIC still plastic. Place *composite* in 2–3 mm increments in stacked angles from base outwards, light curing each increment (20 s). Ensure uncured monomer of the oxygen-inhibited layer on surface of each increment is undisturbed to allow adhesion of next increment. Shape occlusal morphology.	Remove rubber dam. *GIC:* wait 3 min for initial set. Check margins/occlusion with articulating paper. Final occlusal adjustments made with diamond burs/stones/sharp scalpel blade. Finish with diamond polishing paste and coat with lightly filled resin for GIC surface protection (dry surface, paint on resin and light cure (470 nm, 20 s)). *Composites:* Finish surface morphology/margins with fine diamond burs/discs, check margins/occlusion with articulating paper, polish using diamond grit-impregnated cups/discs.

Figure 7.4
(b) Preoperative view of the occlusal surface of LR7 (mICDAS 2). Rubber dam isolation in place, held anteriorly with medium wedget (yellow).

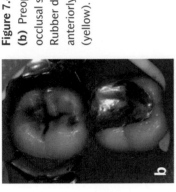

Figure 7.4
(d) 330 TC bur in air-turbine handpiece used to gain enamel access. Rose-head bur in slow-speed handpiece and excavators used to remove caries-infected dentine.

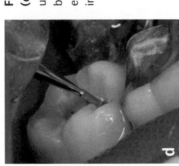

Figure 7.4
(f,g) Silorane primer rubbed onto cavity surfaces (10 s) using a micro-brush, air-thinned for 5 s and light cured (470 nm, 20 s).

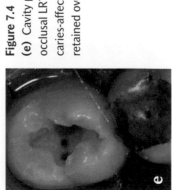

Figure 7.4
(a) Right bitewing radiograph showing multiple early enamel lesions in a high risk patient.

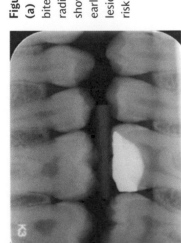

Figure 7.4
(c) Operating view showing rubber dam cut away from nose with paper towel beneath (white). Note operator's finger rests on lower incisors.

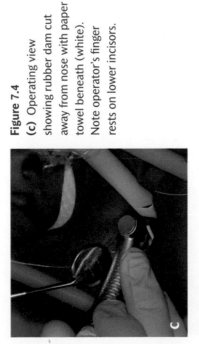

Figure 7.4
(e) Cavity preparation occlusal LR7, with caries-affected dentine retained over pulp.

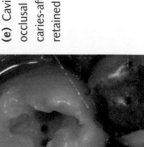

7

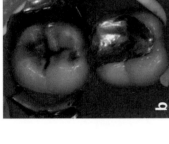

Figure 7.4 (j,k) Silorane composite placed directly into cavity and adapted using pear-shaped burnishers.

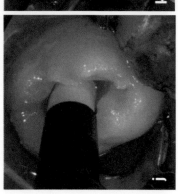

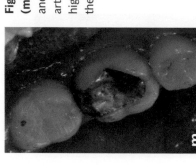

Figure 7.4 (m) Rubber dam removed and occlusion checked with articulating paper – note the high spot marked in red on the distal aspect LR7.

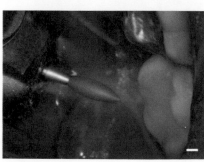

Figure 7.4 (p) Final silorane (low-shrink composite) restoration LR7.

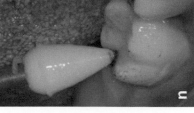

7

Figure 7.4 (h,i) Viscous silorane adhesive rubbed onto cavity surfaces for 10 s, air-thinned for 5 s. And finally light cured (470 nm, 20 s).

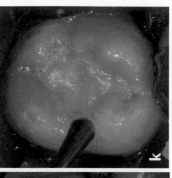

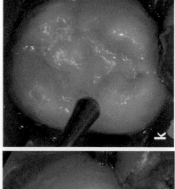

Figure 7.4 (l) Occlusal composite adjusted using fine diamond rugby ball shaped bur.

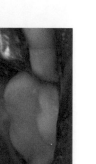

Figure 7.4 (n,o) High spot removed/restoration finished using silica-impregnated points/cups. Note how the finishing point has blunted in use. More pressure increases abrasiveness of point but increases wear on the bur.

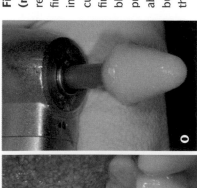

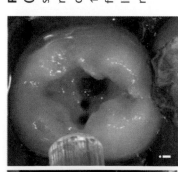

7

7.5　Posterior proximal adhesive restoration (Class II)

Table 7.5 Operative procedure: posterior proximal adhesive restoration (Class II)

Operative procedure 7.5	Indication (Chapters 2,3)	Preoperative procedures/ isolation (Chapter 5)	Caries removal/ cavity preparation (Chapter 5)	Cavity modification (Chapter 5)	Bonding steps (Chapter 6)	Restorative steps	Finishing steps
Posterior proximal adhesive restoration (Class II) Contact point present. If approximal lesion directly accessible by instruments (e.g. no adjacent contact, rotated tooth), then treat as buccal cervical restoration (see Table 7.6).	Approximal cavitated lesion/ mICDAS 3,4. PA radiograph to ascertain depth; pulp response to sensibility tests.	Check occlusion with articulating paper, preoperatively. Select tooth – material shade (Vita guides). Place rubber dam. Pre-wedge adjacent teeth to aid rubber dam placement. Ensure dam can be placed and held firmly cervical to the base of the carious lesion (clamps, wedgets, floss).	Remove unsupported enamel with TC/diamond bur (air-turbine) accessing approximal lesion through occlusal surface, just medial to the relevant marginal ridge. Once access gained to approximal infected dentine, remove undermined marginal ridge with excavator or bur. Peripheral dentine caries excavation (CS bur, hand excavator) to affected/sound dentine (lesion depth, moisture control-dependent) – '**box' preparation.** Excavate infected dentine overlying pulp with hand excavator/avoid exposure. Leave sound enamel periphery, bevelled if possible/avoid gingival papilla trauma.	Wash away debris with water from 3-1 syringe and dry (10 s total). Place sectional/ circumferential metal matrix band interproximally ensuring tight adaptation cervically with wedges and contact point formation. Circumferential band/retainers may interfere with rubber dam clamps.	*Composite:* dependent upon the DBA used (types 1–4, see Table 7.12). GIC (*if difficulty gaining moisture control*): 10% polyacrylic acid conditioner rubbed onto cavity walls with micro-brush (15 s), wash and dry (10 s).	Place *composite* in 2–3 mm increments in stacked angles from base of box outwards, adapting against walls and matrix band, light curing each increment (470 nm, 20 s). Ensure uncured monomer of the oxygen-inhibited layer on the surface of each cured increment is uncontaminated allowing adhesion of next increment. Shape occlusal morphology with carving instruments. Mix/dispense GIC into box base upwards (prevent voids/improve adaptation to cavity walls). Slightly overfill cavity. After 60 s pack GIC into cavity with burnishers/flat plastics ensuring adequate condensation. Occlusal morphology adapted with flat plastics.	Remove rubber dam. *Composites:* Finish composite surface with fine diamond burs/ discs/interproximal finishing strips, check margins/occlusion with articulating paper, polish using diamond grit-impregnated cups/discs. *GIC:* wait 3–4 min for initial set. Check margins/occlusion with articulating paper. Adjustments made with diamond burs/stones/sharp scalpel blade. Finish with diamond polishing paste and coat with lightly filled resin for GIC surface protection.

7.5.1 Posterior proximal adhesive restoration (Class II), type 3 DBA (enamel pre-etch)

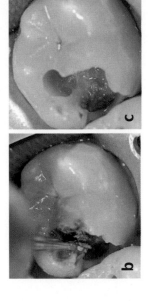

Figure 7.5

(a) Cavitated LR8 with mesio-occlusal caries (mICDAS 4) and a lesion present in the distal-occlusal pit (mICDAS 2), both requiring operative intervention. Tooth isolated with rubber dam using a steel wingless molar clamp (threaded with dental floss to enable retrieval in case the clamp dislodges from tooth or fractures).

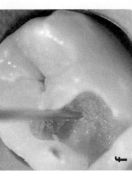 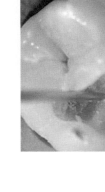

Figure 7.5

(b,c) Using a 330 bur in an air-turbine handpiece, access to dentine caries is improved by removing grossly unsupported and undermined enamel at the cavity margins.

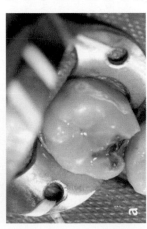

Figure 7.5

(d) Size 3 rose-head carbon steel bur in a slow-speed handpiece removing peripheral caries at the EDJ.

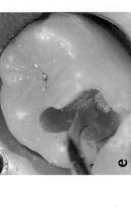

Figure 7.5

(e) Pulpal caries-infected dentine (soft and wet) is carefully removed using a spoon excavator.

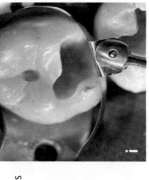

Figure 7.5

(f) The cavity floor is scratchy and flaky, indicative of caries-affected dentine over the pulp.

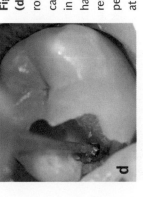

Figure 7.5

(g) The enamel margin at the base of the mesial box can then be finished using a gingival margin trimmer.

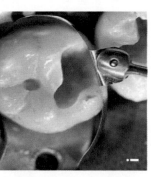

Figure 7.5

(h) The enamel margins are lightly bevelled using a multifluted tungsten carbide bur. Note how the distal occlusal pit lesion has been accessed in a similar fashion to the preventive resin restoration.

Figure 7.5

(i) Placing the sectional metal matrix band in order to reconstitute the mesial wall of the restoration (see Chapter 5). The precurved, contoured band is worked interproximally.

7

7

Figure 7.5
(l) Oval retainer with curved tines, placed to secure and adapt band to LR8: this is checked using a sharp dental explorer at the base of the mesial box, ensuring there is no space through which restorative material can extrude.

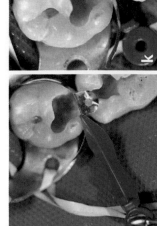

Figure 7.5
(j,k) Gingivally contoured plastic wedge is selected and inserted buccally to maintain tight adaptation of band to the mesial surface of LR8.

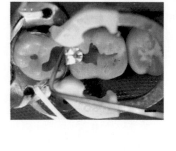

Figure 7.5
(o) Air-dried for 5 s to evaporate solvent carrier, until there is no 'rippling' of the primer film on tooth surface.

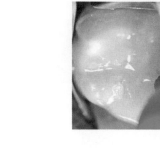

Figure 7.5
(n) Self-etching primer (type 3 DBA) is rubbed onto the cavity walls for 10 s.

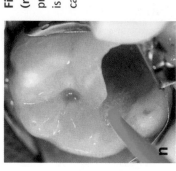

Figure 7.5
(m) Enamel margins pre-etched with 37% orthophosphoric acid etch gel for 15 s, washed off for 10 s, and gently air-dried for 2–3 s.

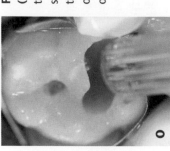

Figure 7.5
(r) Occlusal cavity restored with flowable composite. Dentine shade resin composite directly introduced into the mesiolingual aspect of the cavity LR8.

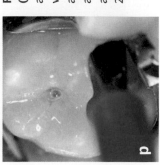

Figure 7.5
(q) This results in shiny cavity surfaces which must be present prior to placing the first increment of resin composite.

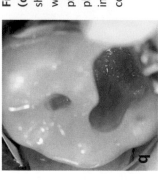

Figure 7.5
(p) Type 3 bond is applied to cavity walls for 10 s, air-thinned using 3-1 air/water syringe and light cured for 20 s (470 nm).

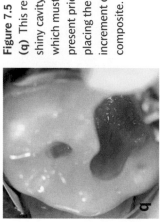

Figure 7.5
(u,v) Final increments are placed, adapted and light cured, leaving space for the enamel shade composite to be placed.

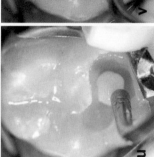
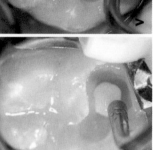

Figure 7.5
(t) Further 2 mm increments placed and adapted to form the mesial wall of the restoration against firm matrix band and light cured.

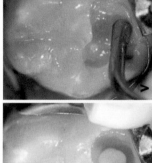

Figure 7.5
(s) Increment is adapted using a pear-shaped burnisher and then light cured for 20 s (470 nm).

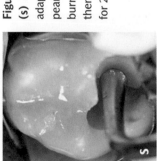

Figure 7.5
(w) Using Ward's/Half-Hollenback carver, occlusal morphology introduced in the enamel composite, including mesial marginal ridge, fossae, and fissure pattern.

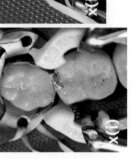

Figure 7.5
(x) Retainer removed with clamp, wedge removed buccally, and sectional matrix teased from interproximal area using special tweezers.

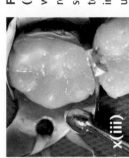
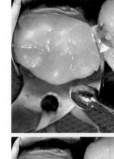
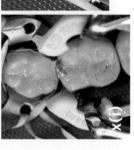

Figure 7.5
(y) Fine diamond grit/multifluted tungsten carbide burs are used to adjust the occlusal/axial surfaces of the restoration after checking the occlusion with articulating paper. Proximal surfaces finished with strips/checked with floss.

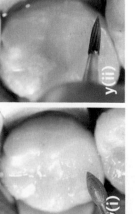
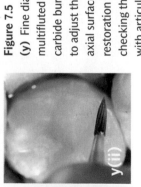

Figure 7.5
(z) Composite surface then finished using silica-impregnated cups and points of reducing coarseness. Diamond polishing pastes can help achieve a high lustre. Final restoration.

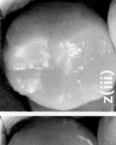
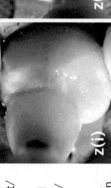

7

7

7.5.2 Posterior proximal adhesive restoration (Class II), type 2 DBA, 'moist bonding'

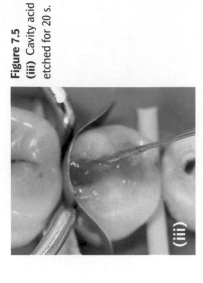

Figure 7.5 (iii) Cavity acid etched for 20 s.

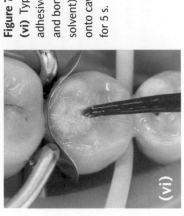
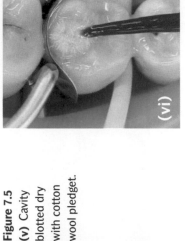

Figure 7.5 (i,ii) LR5 distal-occlusal cavity (Class II), isolated with rubber dam (wingless clamp LL7 and medium wedget, mesial LL5). Sectional matrix band, wedged gingivally and retained with oval ring.

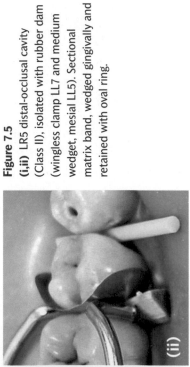

Figure 7.5 (vi) Type 2 adhesive (primer and bond plus solvent) rubbed onto cavity walls for 5 s.

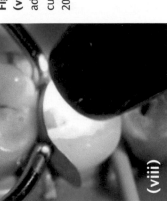

Figure 7.5 (v) Cavity blotted dry with cotton wool pledget.

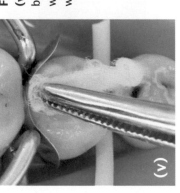

Figure 7.5 (viii) Type 2 adhesive light cured (470nm, 20 s).

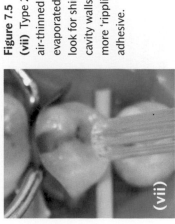

Figure 7.5 (iv) Cavity washed for 10 s.

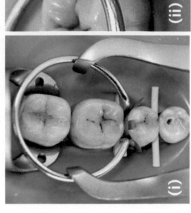

Figure 7.5 (vii) Type 2 adhesive air-thinned and solvent evaporated for 5 s – look for shiny film on cavity walls and no more 'rippling' of adhesive.

Figure 7.5
(ix,x) Resin composite placed and adapted into distal box using pear-shaped burnisher. Increments light cured.

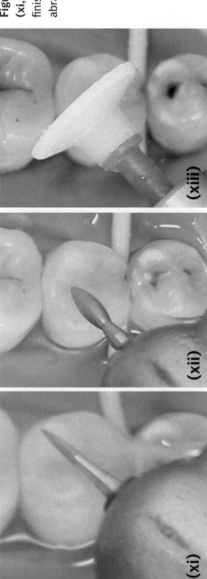

(ix) (x)

Figure 7.5
(xi,xii,xiii) Resin composite trimmed and finished using fine diamond finishing burs and abrasive polishing discs.

(xi) (xii) (xiii)

Figure 7.5
(xiv, xv) Resin composite finished proximally using abrasive finishing strip, ensuring good distal contour to the final restoration.

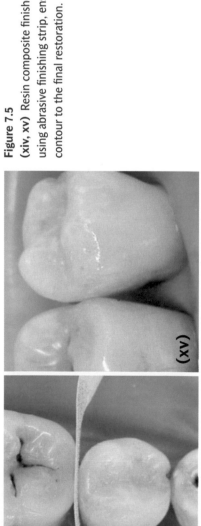

(xiv) (xv)

7

7

7.6 Buccal cervical resin composite restorations (Class V), type 2 DBA

Table 7.6 Operative procedure: buccal cervical resin composite restoration

Operative procedure 7.6	Indication (Chapters 2,3)	Preoperative procedures/ isolation (Chapter 5)	Caries removal/ cavity preparation (Chapter 5)	Cavity modification (Chapter 5)	Bonding steps (Chapter 6)	Restorative steps	Finishing steps
Buccal/ lingual cervical adhesive restoration (Class V)	Discoloured anterior/ posterior toothwear (causing plaque stagnation or risk of structural weakness). Cavitated carious lesion/ mICDAS 3,4/ pulp response?	Select tooth – material shade. Moisture control: rubber dam isolation often difficult as clamp/dam obscures access to lesion margins. Simpler cotton wool isolation/ aspiration may be necessary.	Caries: remove unsupported and/or undermined demineralized enamel with TC/ diamond bur (air-turbine). Leave sound enamel margin (may be difficult cervically). Peripheral dentine caries excavation (CS bur, hand excavator) to affected/sound dentine (lesion depth dependent). Avoid gingival trauma. Excavate infected dentine overlying pulp with hand excavator/avoid exposure. Toothwear lesion: ideally air-abrade exposed lesion surface, removing stain and surface debris.	Lightly bevel sound enamel margins using fine diamond bur, air-turbine. Wash away debris with water from 3-1 syringe and dry (10 s total).	*Composite:* dependent upon the DBA used (types 1–4, see Table 7.12). *GIC (if difficulty gaining moisture control):* 10% polyacrylic acid conditioner rubbed onto cavity walls with micro-brush (15 s), wash and dry (10 s).	Place *composite* in 2–3 mm increments in stacked angles base of cavity outwards, light curing each increment (470 nm, 20 s). Shape occlusal morphology with flat plastic instruments or cervical matrices, removing excess prior to curing. Mix/dispense *GIC* filling from base up (prevent voids). Slightly overfill cavity. After 60 s adapt GIC with burnishers/flat plastics to ensure adequate condensation. Surface may be adapted using cervical matrices.	*Composites:* Remove rubber dam. Finish composite surface morphology/margins with fine diamond burs/discs, check margins and polish using diamond grit-impregnated cups/discs. *GIC:* wait 3–4 min for initial set. Final contour adjusted with diamond burs/ stones/sharp scalpel blade. Finish with diamond polishing paste and coat with lightly filled resin for GIC surface protection.

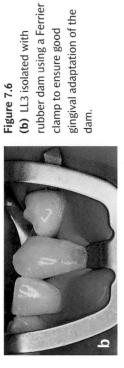

Figure 7.6
(a) Buccal cervical cavity LL3 with plaque stagnation. Gingival margin finishing on dentine.

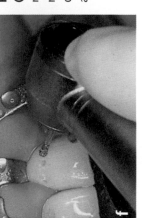

Figure 7.6
(b) LL3 isolated with rubber dam using a Ferrier clamp to ensure good gingival adaptation of the dam.

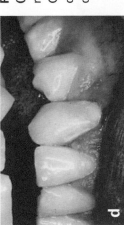

Figure 7.6
(c) Acid-etch gel placed on all cavity surfaces for 20 s, washed off (10 s) and air-dried for 2–3 s ('moist bonding' – no enamel frosting visible). Adhesive then rubbed onto cavity, air-thinned for 5 s, checked for shiny film and light cured (470 nm, 20 s).

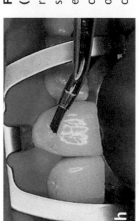

Figure 7.6
(d) Final buccal cervical restoration placed in LL3. Contour achieved using diamond finishing burs and discs.

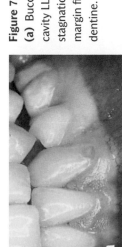

Figure 7.6
(e) Two small enamel pits on the labial surface UL1 causing an aesthetic concern.

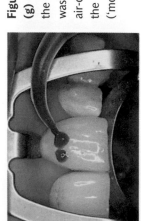

Figure 7.6
(f) Teeth isolated with rubber dam and stain removed with a round diamond bur in the air-turbine handpiece.

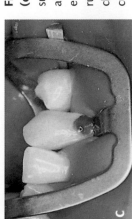

Figure 7.6
(g) Acid-etch gel placed on the enamel cavities for 20 s, washed off for 10 s and air-dried for 2–3 s to remove the surface water droplets ('moist bonding').

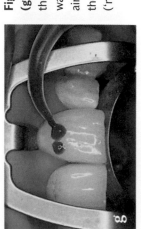

Figure 7.6
(h) Type 2 adhesive rubbed onto the cavity surfaces, air-thinned to evaporate solvent (5 s) and checked for the presence of a shiny film, then light cured.

7

7

Figure 7.6 (k) Composite light cured – note the orange filter held in front of the light to protect the nurse's and operator's eyes from the intense 470 nm light.

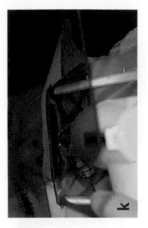

Figure 7.6 (i,j) Flowable resin composite (shade checked before rubber dam placement) dispensed into cavities and adapted using a titanium nitride-coated non-stick carver.

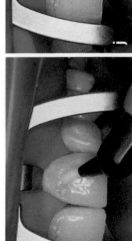

Figure 7.6 (m) UL1 restoration finished using fine abrasive discs.

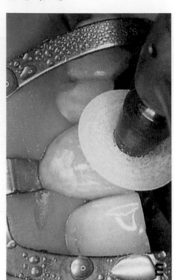

Figure 7.6 (l) Composite adjusted using fine diamond burs with a water spray.

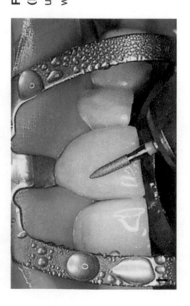

Figure 7.6 (n) Final restoration UL1.

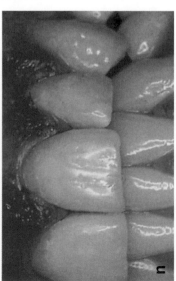

7

7.7 Anterior proximal adhesive restoration (Class III), type 2 DBA

Table 7.7 Operative procedure: anterior proximal adhesive restoration

Operative procedure 7.7	Indication (Chapters 2,3)	Preoperative procedures/ isolation (Chapter 5)	Caries removal/cavity preparation (Chapter 5)	Cavity modification (Chapter 5)	Bonding steps (Chapter 6)	Restorative steps	Finishing steps
Anterior proximal adhesive restoration (Class III)	Cavitated carious lesion/ mICDAS 3,4/ pulp response/ plaque stagnation. Replacement of discoloured/ failed restoration.	Check palatal guiding occlusion with articulating paper, preoperatively. Select tooth – material shade (Vita guides – dentine/ enamel shades). Place rubber dam. Pre-wedge adjacent teeth to aid rubber dam placement. Ensure dam can be placed and held firmly cervical to the base of the carious lesion (clamps, wedgets, floss).	Caries: remove unsupported/ undermined demineralized enamel with TC/diamond bur from palatal aspect (air-turbine). Preserve labial enamel wall if possible to aid aesthetics. Leave sound enamel margin (may be difficult cervically). Peripheral dentine caries excavation (CS bur, hand excavator) to affected/sound dentine (lesion depth dependent). Avoid gingival trauma. Excavate infected dentine overlying pulp with hand excavator/avoid exposure.	Lightly bevel sound enamel margins using fine diamond bur, air-turbine. Wash away debris with water from 3-1 syringe and dry (10 s total). Place 15 mm long, clear matrix strip interproximally and wedge cervically (contact point, cervical adaptation of restorative material).	*Composite:* dependent upon the DBA used (types 1–4, see Table 7.12).	Place *composite* in 2–3 mm increments in stacked angles from base of cavity outwards, light curing each increment (470 nm, 20 s). Consider aesthetic layering techniques with dentine and enamel shades. Ensure uncured monomer of the oxygen-inhibited layer on the surface of each cured increment is uncontaminated prior to placement of the next to allow adhesion of next increment. Shape palatal morphology with flat plastic instruments, removing excess prior to curing.	Remove wedge, clear matrix band and rubber dam. Finish composite surface morphology/ margins with fine diamond burs/discs/ interproximal finishing strips. Check margins with probe/ protrusive guiding occlusion with articulating paper. Polish using diamond grit-impregnated cups/discs.

**Figure 7.7
(b)** The same lesion on UL1; note palatal shadowing.

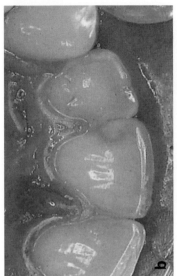

**Figure 7.7
(a)** Anterior view of a proximal carious lesion (mICDAS 2) on the distal surface of UL1.

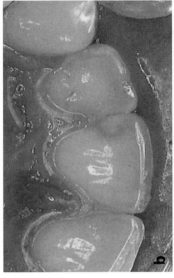

**Figure 7.7
(d)** Shows the enamel distal marginal ridge cleared through the contact area with the adjacent UL2. Note the brown dentine caries still present.

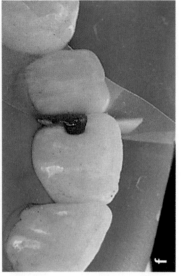

**Figure 7.7
(c)** Palatal access cut through enamel using a small round bur in the air-turbine handpiece.

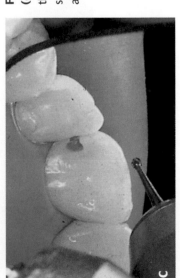

**Figure 7.7
(f)** Clear plastic strip is placed interproximally and wedged against the tooth surface. The cavity is etched for 20 s using 37% orthophosphoric acid etch.

**Figure 7.7
(e)** All stained dentine excavated leaving yellow hard sound dentine at cavity base for aesthetic reasons, preventing shadowing beneath the final restoration. Labial enamel is preserved.

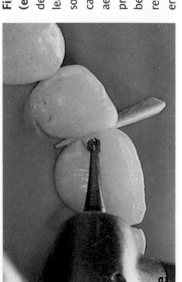

7

7

Figure 7.7
(h) Dentine/enamel resin composite placed incrementally and light cured. Palatal surface contour smoothed with rugby ball shaped fine diamond composite finishing bur. Occlusion checked with articulating paper.

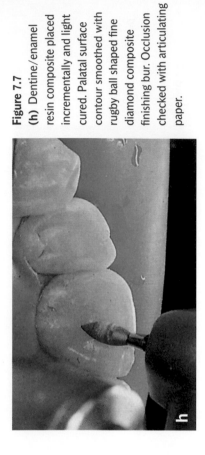

Figure 7.7
(g) Etch is rinsed away (10 s) and dried with cotton pledgets ('moist bond technique') before applying the dentine bonding agent and light curing for 20 s.

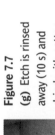

Figure 7.7
(j) Final Class III distal restoration UL1.

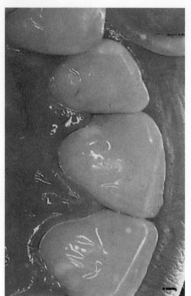

Figure 7.7
(i) Proximal surface finished using abrasive finishing strip (coarse then fine), taking care to preserve the contact point.

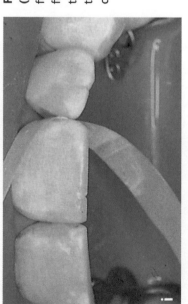

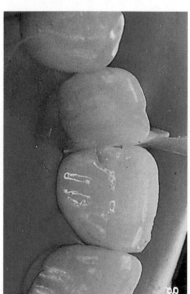
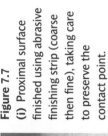

7

7.8 Anterior incisal edge/labial composite veneer (Class IV), type 3 DBA (enamel pre-etch)

Table 7.8 Operative procedure: anterior incisal edge/labial composite veneer

Operative procedure 7.8	Indication (Chapters 2,3)	Preoperative procedures/isolation (Chapter 5)	Caries removal/cavity preparation (Chapter 5)	Cavity modification (Chapter 5)	Bonding steps (Chapter 6)	Restorative steps	Finishing steps
Anterior incisal edge (Class IV) **Direct veneer restoration**	Replacement of discoloured/failed restoration. Traumatic fracture of coronal enamel/dentine. Aesthetic masking of intrinsic staining, minor alteration of labial morphology. Toothwear lesions caries – high risk patients.	Check palatal/protrusive guiding occlusion with articulating paper, preoperatively. Select tooth – material shade (Vita guides – dentine/enamel shades depending on the composite system). Place rubber dam. Pre-wedge adjacent teeth to aid rubber dam placement. Ensure dam can be placed and held firmly cervical to the base of the carious lesion (clamps, wedgets, floss).	Remove old composite restoration with diamond/TC bur, air-turbine or bioactive glass/alumina air-abrasion. Excavate soft caries-infected and stained caries-affected dentine with excavators/CS rose-head burs. Remove extrinsic staining with sodium bicarbonate air-polishing, bioactive glass air-abrasion. Achieve sound enamel margins at periphery of cavity.	Long, undulated bevel cut into sound enamel on labial surface, fine long-tapered diamond bur, air-turbine. Short bevel placed on the palatal aspect. Sharp line angles rounded off. Wash away debris with water from 3-1 syringe and dry (10 s total). Place 15 mm-long clear matrix strip interproximally and wedge cervically.	Composite: dependent on the DBA used (types 1–4, see Table 7.12).	Place composite in 2–3 mm increments in stacked angles from palatal aspect of cavity labially, light curing each (470 nm, 20 s). Can use preformed rigid acrylic/putty matrix outlining the palatal contour, incisal/mesial/distal margins; interproximal strips cannot be used with matrices. Consider aesthetic layering techniques with dentine and enamel shades. Ensure uncured monomer of the oxygen-inhibited layer on the surface of each cured increment is uncontaminated to allow adhesion of next increment. Shape morphology with Ward's/Half-Hollenback carver removing excess.	Remove wedge, clear matrix band and rubber dam. Finish composite surface morphology/margins with fine diamond burs/discs/interproximal finishing strips. Check margins with probe/protrusive guiding occlusion with articulating paper. Polish using diamond grit-impregnated cups/discs.

Figure 7.8

(a) UL1 mesioincisal enamel–dentine fracture (Class IV) causing sensitivity and an aesthetic concern.

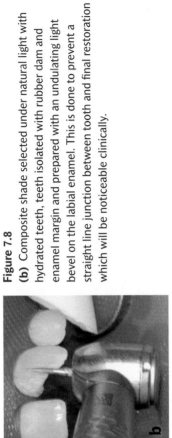
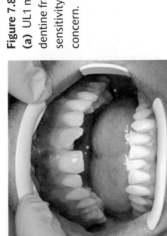
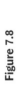

Figure 7.8

(b) Composite shade selected under natural light with hydrated teeth, teeth isolated with rubber dam and enamel margin and prepared with an undulating light bevel on the labial enamel. This is done to prevent a straight line junction between tooth and final restoration which will be noticeable clinically.

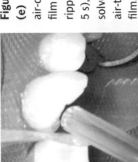

Figure 7.8

(c) Acid-etch gel placed all over enamel margins and labial enamel for 20 s, washed and dried (10 s).

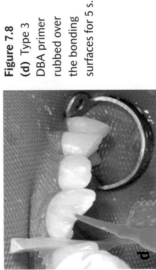

Figure 7.8

(d) Type 3 DBA primer rubbed over the bonding surfaces for 5 s.

Figure 7.8

(e) Primer air-dried until film no longer ripples (approx. 5 s), removing solvent and air-thinning the film.

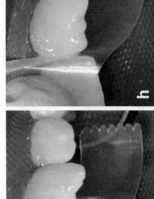

Figure 7.8

(f) Type 3 DBA bond rubbed over the cavity surfaces for 5 s, and air-thinned as before and light cured.

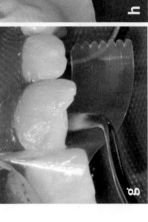
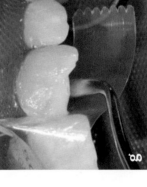

Figure 7.8

(g,h) Dentine shade composite placed to form the palatal wall of the final restoration. Note how the clear matrix strip is wedge cervically for marginal adaptation. The underlying mammelon anatomy is mimicked with the composite. This is light cured (470 nm, 20 s).

7

7

Figure 7.8 (j,k) Roll of enamel shade composite is then teased cervically across the labial surface with the flat plastic, thinning as it blends with the natural tooth along the undulating bevel.

k

j

Figure 7.8 (i) Enamel composite is placed as a roll along the incisal edge of UL1 using a flat plastic.

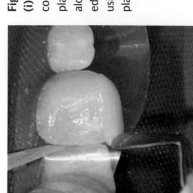

i

Figure 7.8 (m,n) Margins are trimmed using composite finishing fine diamond burs cervically, proximally and palatally (rugby ball shaped bur).

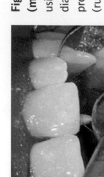

n

m

Figure 7.8 (l) This process permits the placement of a smooth homogenous layer of composite labially, that is easily finished later.

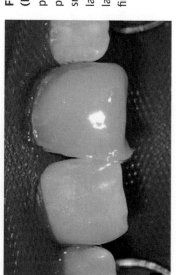

l

Figure 7.8 (q) This is removed using a fine diamond bur.

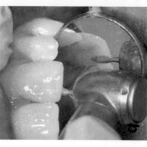

q

Figure 7.8 (o,p) Incisal occlusion is assessed using articulating paper. Finger placed on UL1 to 'feel' the heavy contact – *fremitus*. A heavy contact is expressed on the mesiopalatal aspect of UL1, with the straight line trace of the protrusive guidance (towards the incisal edge).

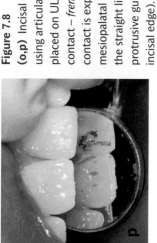

p

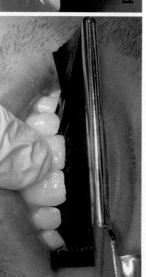

o

Figure 7.8 (r,s,t) The teeth are dried with cotton wool rolls and the occlusion rechecked this time showing a light contact distocervically UL1 – normal incisal contact.

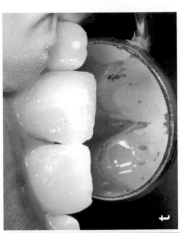

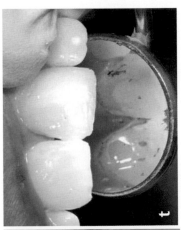

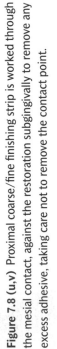

Figure 7.8 (w,x) Composite polished with coarse to fine abrasive points and discs, achieving a final high surface lustre and surface anatomy.

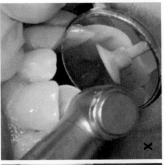
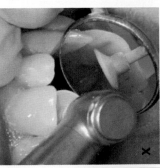
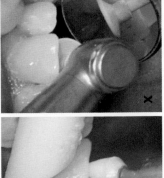

Figure 7.8 (u,v) Proximal coarse/fine finishing strip is worked through the mesial contact, against the restoration subgingivally to remove any excess adhesive, taking care not to remove the contact point.

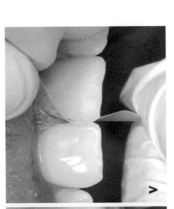

Figure 7.8 (y) Final aesthetic composite restoration UL1 with the patient smiling. Note the final shade seems slightly darker than the adjacent natural dentition – this is due to dehydration of the natural teeth making them appear whiter. The patient should be warned about this prior to starting the procedure. This will correct itself within a few hours.

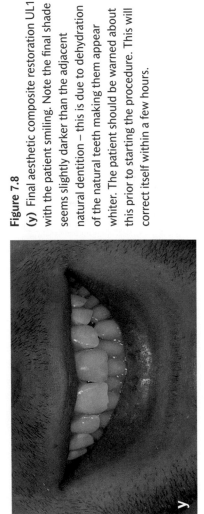

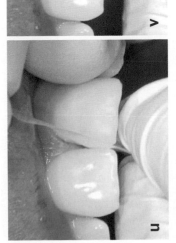

7

7.9 Large posterior amalgam restoration (bonded) (courtesy of Dr G Palmer)

Table 7.9 Operative procedure: large posterior amalgam restoration

Operative procedure 7.9	Indication (Chapters 2,3)	Preoperative procedures/ isolation (Chapter 5)	Caries removal/ cavity preparation (Chapter 5)	Cavity modification (Chapter 5)	Bonding steps (Chapter 6)	Restorative steps	Finishing steps
Large posterior amalgam restoration	Heavily broken down coronal tooth structure. High load-bearing, large restoration. Core build up for posterior root-filled teeth. Difficult moisture control conditions.	Check occlusion preoperatively with articulating paper. Cotton wool rolls/ aspiration or rubber dam isolation if possible.	Cavity/defect already present – access cavity from endodontic treatment, fractured cusps. Caries – biologically excavate to sound dentine using hand excavators/CS rose-head burs. Remove undermined/ unsupported enamel (diamond/TC burs, air-turbine).	Undercut dentine at diametrically opposite aspects of cavity (CS rose-head bur), if remaining tissue permits this. Round off sharp internal line angles. Smooth cavity base. Indirect pulp capping over blushing pulp with GIC. Wash away debris and dry (10 s). Place circumferential matrix band, wedging the cervical aspect interproximally.	*Bonded amalgams:* use auto-/dual-cure resin cement (e.g. Panavia F2).	Triturate high-Cu alloy, plug and condense incrementally from the base of the cavity outwards, ensuring adaptation against walls/matrix. Slightly overfill cavity and carve back to occlusal level and morphology using carvers (Ward's, Half-Hollenback), flat plastics. Work quickly but not hastily!	Remove matrix band. Take care not to fracture/dislodge marginal ridges. Check occlusion with articulating paper/interproximal overhangs with dental floss/finishing abrasive strips. Remove high spots with excavator/Mitchell's trimmer or amalgam finishing burs if required. Burnish occlusal surface and margins for smooth finish and good adaptation. Wipe occlusal surface with slightly damp cotton wool pledget for final surface finish.

Figure 7.9

(b) Circumferential metal matrix band with retainer placed around tooth and wedged distolingually using a wooden wedge to help adaptation of the distal margin of the final restoration. The band's inner surface is lightly coated with petroleum jelly to aid its final removal. To aid retention, a self-etching primer has been rubbed onto the cavity surface and air-dried to thin and evaporate the solvent.

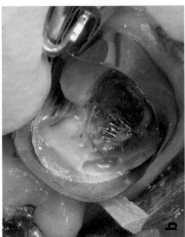

Figure 7.9

(d) The amalgam is condensed into the cavity, filling the volume of the matrix band while keeping in mind the cuspal height of the adjacent teeth. The excess amalgam has been removed around the margins (yellow arrows) so exposing the edge of the band.

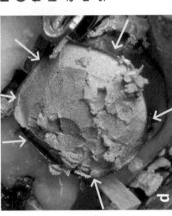

Figure 7.9

(f) Using the curved blade of a sickle scaler, the buccal and lingual walls of the amalgam are contoured, closely following that of the adjacent teeth. The height of the amalgam is reduced to the level of the final cusp tips.

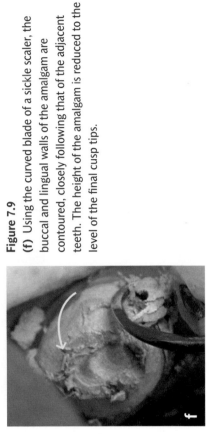

Figure 7.9

(a) Grossly broken down LL6 prepared for an amalgam restoration. Note the two lingual slots (green arrows) and relative undercuts around the mesiobuccal cusp to aid retention (black arrows) and the distobuccal heavy shoulder preparation to aid distal support (white arrow).

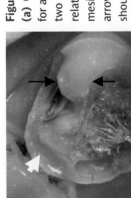

Figure 7.9

(c) A thin chemically cured resin adhesive cement applied using a microbrush onto the cavity surfaces – this technique is known as a bonded amalgam, assisting retention in very large cavities.

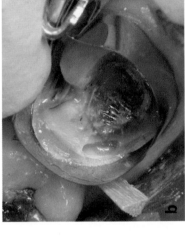

Figure 7.9

(e) After a few minutes, the wedge is removed, band loosened and pushed sideways lingually, through the contact area (note the gap, arrowed). The amalgam is supported with a Guy's pattern plugger as the matrix band is eased off.

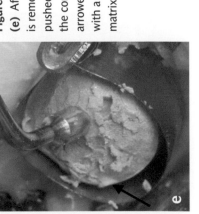

7

7

Figure 7.9

(h) Using a Half-Hollenback or Ward's carver, carve in the central fissure pattern (blue line) by joining up the three fossae (green dots). To maintain cusp bulk, try to carve from the fossae up to the transverse ridge (purple lines) and then back down to the adjacent fossa.

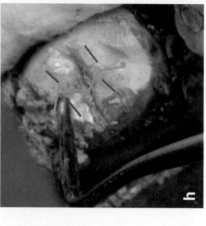

Figure 7.9

(j) After checking the occlusion and margins, the final restoration is burnished and a smooth surface achieved by gently rubbing the surface with a damp cotton wool pledget. Courtesy Dr. G. Palmer.

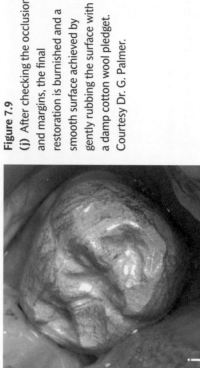

Figure 7.9

(g) The mesial and distal marginal ridges are carved to the height of the adjacent ridges, followed by the marginal ridge and central fossae using a spoon excavator.

Figure 7.9

(i) Refine the final occlusal morphology and anatomy using carvers (Ward's or Half-Hollenback), sickle scaler, excavator, and/or Mitchell's trimmer and check occlusion using articulating paper.

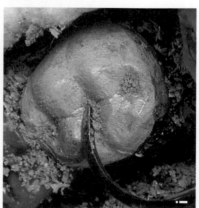

7

7.10 'Nayyar core' restoration

Table 7.10 Operative procedure: 'Nayyar core' restoration

Operative procedure 7.10	Indication (Chapters 2,3)	Preoperative procedures/ isolation (Chapter 5)	Caries removal/cavity preparation (Chapter 5)	Cavity modification (Chapter 5)	Bonding steps (Chapter 6)	Restorative steps	Finishing steps
'Nayyar core' restoration Amalgam GIC Composite	Posterior root-filled teeth with short, curved root canals. Enough cervical coronal dentine must remain to support the final restoration. Technique provides retention and strength for the coronal restoration.	Rubber dam isolation if possible. Cotton wool rolls/aspiration.	Use already created endodontic access cavity and natural shape of the pulp chamber. Remove coronal 2–4 mm of root-canal filling (e.g. gutta percha) from the obturated canals, using Gates-Glidden burs.	Remove any sharp internal line angles with CS rose-head bur. Wash and dry final cavity (10 s). Place suitable matrix as required to replace any missing coronal walls of cavity.	*Bonded amalgam:* auto-/dual-cure resin cement. *GIC:* 10% polyacrylic acid conditioner, 15 s (wash and dry, 10 s). *Composite:* DBA, types 1–4 (Table 7.12). Original Nayyar core described using dental amalgam, but adhesive materials may be used with their own bonding procedures.	Triturate, plug and condense amalgam into the openings created in the coronal aspect of the root canals using narrow Smith plugger/periodontal probe. Pack the remaining cavity, slight overfill and carve back using appropriate carvers. For composites/ GICs – ensure the root canal spaces are filled without voids, using a dark shade. Place fine capsule tips into canal orifice and back fill (GIC). Light cure composite increments (470 nm, 20 s).	Remove rubber dam/ matrix band. Check interproximal margins with floss and remove overhangs/finish surfaces with amalgam/composite finishing strips. Check occlusion with articulating paper and adjust high spots with carvers/ amalgam burs (amalgam), fine diamond burs/discs (GIC/composite). Burnish final amalgam/finish with diamond-impregnated polishing discs (GIC/composite).

7.11 Direct fibre-post/composite core restoration

Table 7.11 Operative procedure: direct fibre-post/composite core restoration

Operative procedure 7.11	Indication (Chapters 2,3)	Preoperative procedures/ isolation (Chapter 5)	Caries removal/ cavity preparation (Chapter 5)	Cavity modification (Chapter 5)	Bonding steps (Chapter 6)	Restorative steps	Finishing steps
Direct fibre-post/ composite core restoration	Broken down anterior (and posterior) root-filled teeth. Relatively straight root canal(s). Technique retains large adhesive coronal restoration and may reinforce remaining coronal/ radicular tooth structure.	PA radiograph of root-filled tooth. Choose shade of composite. Rubber dam isolation ideally.	Remove gutta percha root filling using Gates-Glidden burs. Calculate radicular post length from original length of post minus the length of post required coronally. Take into account root canal length, ensuring a minimum of 4 mm gutta percha is retained apically. Use LCPA radiograph. Gauge diameter of post from PA radiograph. Prepare post hole using supplied post drills (narrow-wide diameter in stages). Wash and dry post hole (paper points). Holding fibre-reinforced post with college tweezers, try post in for size and fit. Section post to required length (if necessary) using a carborundum disc, from coronal end.	Round off any sharp line angles on the coronal surface. Wash post hole with NaOCl and dry with paper points. Clean fibre-post with alcohol and air-dry for 5 s.	Use self-etching dual-cure resin cement (e.g. RelyX Unicem (3MESPE)). Activate capsule, automix, attach fine nozzle and backfill post hole.	Insert fibre-post, hold in place, remove excess cement with flat plastic instrument and light cure (470 nm, 40 s) or wait 5 min. Apply DBA (types 1–4 – Table 7.12) on to coronal tooth surface and coronal portion of post. Place interproximal clear matrix strips to separate adjacent teeth/ help create contact points. Incrementally place composite, building up dentine/enamel shades if chosen, to provisionalize tooth. Start around post, light cure (470 nm) for 20 s and layer next increment. Ensure post is covered with composite.	Remove rubber dam/matrix strips. Check approximal margins with floss – smooth with composite finishing strips. Check occlusion with articulating paper and adjust with fine diamond bur, air-turbine/ discs. Smooth/polish with diamond-impregnated cups/ points/discs.

7

7.12 Dentine bonding agents – step-by-step practical guide

Table 7.12 Dentine bonding agents – types, constituents, and practical tips for clinical use

Type	Smear layer	Etch	Primer	Bond
1 **Three-step** Total etch/ etch and rinse	Remove	37% orthophosphoric acid gel painted on enamel (20 s) and dentine (15 s). Removes smear layer, demineralizes (microporosities in enamel) and exposes dentine collagen fibres. Wash off (10 s) and air-dry (10 s). May notice frosted enamel.	Contains hydrophilic monomer (e.g. HEMA) acting as bi-functional molecules linking hydrophilic collagen to hydrophobic resin monomers, creating the **hybrid layer**. Exists with a carrier – water. Painted on cavity surface with micro-brush (5 s) and gently air-thinned (2–3 s).	Contains HEMA and other, more hydrophobic monomers. Essentially acts as the unfilled (or in some cases, lightly filled) resin composite. This component is painted onto the primer for 5 s and then light cured (470 nm, 20 s). A shiny cavity surface indicates the presence of the cured DBA, ready for first increment of composite.
2 **Two-step** Total etch/ etch and rinse 'moist bonding'	Remove	37% orthophosphoric acid gel painted on enamel (20 s) and dentine (15 s). Removes smear layer, demineralizes (microporosities in enamel) and exposes dentine collagen fibres. Wash off (10 s). Air-dry (2–3 s). Blot away surface water droplets (cotton wool pledgets, paper points) – **moist bonding**. If enamel appears frosted then it is likely the dentine surface is too dry and should be rehydrated.	Primer and bond mixed together in same bottle – known as the 'adhesive'. The more hydrophilic monomer (e.g. HEMA) is carried in a volatile solvent (e.g. acetone or alcohol) easing its penetration into the moist dentine collagen fibres, forming the **hybrid layer**. The combined adhesive is rubbed actively into the cavity surfaces using a micro-brush (5 s). The adhesive is air-dried (5 s) to evaporate the solvent and thin the adhesive layer/prevent pooling within the cavity. Visually check the surface for a 'sheen'; a shiny cavity surface indicates the presence of the adhesive. A dull surface indicates that the adhesive has been blown out of the cavity or has been absorbed into the dentine. If dull, a second layer of adhesive is rubbed in (5 s) and air-dried (5 s) and visually checked. Shiny cavity surfaces can be light cured (470 nm, 20 s) and are then ready for composite.	
3a **Two-step** Weak self-etching primer	Dissolve	The etch and primer have been combined using acidic monomers, creating a self-etching primer. The acidity of these primers is considerably less than that of acid etch. This acidic primer still contains a solvent requiring evaporation, but no washing is required. The acidic primer is applied with the micro-brush on the cavity walls (5 s) and air-dried (5 s), evaporating the solvent/thinning the pooled primer until no rippling of the applied layer is noticed.		The bond has similar chemistry to unfilled/lightly filled resin composite with some hydrophilic monomers included. This adhesive is applied onto the self-etching primer (5 s), air-thinned for 2–3 s and light cured (470 nm, 20 s). A shiny surface appearance indicates the DBA is in place and ready to accept the first increment of composite.
3b **Two-step** Strongly self-etching primer	Dissolve	*Silorane SE Bond (3MESPE)* is a stronger self-etching primer. Applied for 5 s with a micro-brush Air-thin for 2–3 s, visually check for shiny surfaces/no surface rippling Light cured (470 nm, 20 s)		The viscous hydrophobic adhesive bond is then applied with the micro-brush. Light cured (470 nm, 20 s)
4 **One-step** Strong self-etching primer	Dissolve	All-in-one systems that present the three stages (etch, prime, and bond) together in one application. Stronger acidic monomers (e.g. glycerophosphoric acid dimethacrylate) etch the tooth surface, dissolving the smear layer, demineralizing and, in dentine, exposing the collagen fibres to the more hydrophilic monomers to penetrate and form the hybrid layer. DBA premixed and rubbed into the cavity surfaces with a micro-brush (5 s). Air-thinned 2–3 s, visually check for shiny surfaces/no rippling. Light cured (470 nm, 20 s).		

7

7.13 Checking the final restoration

Once any dental restoration has been placed and finished (of varying size, shape and material), it is wise for the operator to get into the habit of running through a final clinical checklist before discharging the patient, evaluating the:

- Occlusion/occlusal morphology/marginal ridge position (assessed using articulating paper pre- and postoperatively)
- Marginal adaptation (positive or negative ledges, overhangs, excess flash material – assessed using straight probe, Briault probe or dental floss approximally)

- Tight contact points (for Class II/III restorations – assessed using dental floss)
- Surface finish (smooth finish assess using a dental probe)
- Aesthetics (especially in the anterior aesthetic zone, colour/translucency co-assessed by the patient).

7.14 Patient instructions

Depending on the type of restorative material used, the patient should be given appropriate instruction on how to look after/manage the new restoration for the immediate 24–48-hour period. In all cases, suitable oral hygiene must be achieved. If local anaesthetic has been used, patients should be warned to take care regarding chewing and biting and consuming hot beverages until the effects have worn off.

- Temporary restorations and amalgam: care must be taken to avoid heavy occlusal loading. Ask the patient to avoid chewing too heavily on the filling.
- Resin composites: no further instruction is required. The patient should have been forewarned of the possible shade changes as the adjacent teeth rehydrate over the few hours immediately after the rubber dam has been removed (Figure 7.8y).

8

Recall, maintenance, and repair

Chapter contents

8.1 Introduction

Dental care involves more than just the operative treatment of the consequences of disease. It concerns controlling/preventing disease (modifying aetiological factors by changes in patient behaviour/attitude) and *monitoring* the oral cavity and restored dentition to ensure that health is *maintained*. Artificial restorations need to be checked regularly and occasionally *repaired* or *replaced* (see Figures 8.1–8.3). Therefore, the recall appointments, once an episode of treatment is completed, are just as important as the direct treatment itself.

Three aspects of dental care to be monitored in recall visits are:

- Quality of the restorations present
- The state of oral and dental health
- The individual patient's longer-term response to previous preventive advice and/or treatment, in moderating any aetiological factors that could cause future dental disease.

8.2 Restoration failure

The potential causes of restoration failure are outlined in Table 8.1. It is important to appreciate that the causes for restoration and tooth failure (Table 8.2) are often multifactorial in nature.

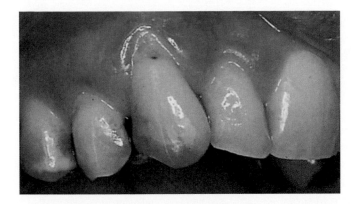

Figure 8.1 Corrosion products from a distal amalgam in the UR3 causing coronal discoloration which the patient complained about, an example of aesthetic restoration failure.

Q8.1: What restorative material should be used to replace this amalgam?

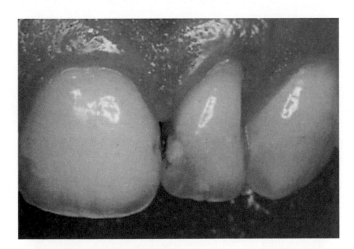

Figure 8.2 An aged, discoloured mesial resin composite restoration on UL2. This provided aesthetic concerns for the patient who requested its replacement.

Q8.2: What would be the difficulty faced by the dentist when replacing this Class III restoration?

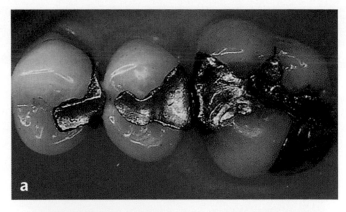

a

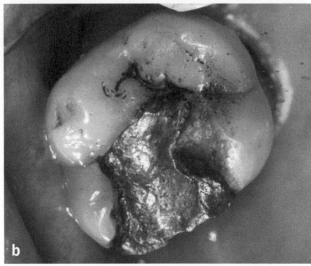

b

Figure 8.3 (**a**) A series of old, ditched and partly corroded amalgam restorations, noticed on clinical examination that these are cleanable and not causing direct problems to the patient. Although the margins and occlusal surfaces are not perfect, are these amalgams classified as failed restorations? (**b**) A ditched amalgam UL7 with marginal space large enough to accommodate the tip of a periodontal probe, accumulating plaque. Replacement in this case would facilitate plaque control.

8

Table 8.1 Causes of restoration failure and the criteria used to assess this failure with clinical comments. It is vital to appreciate that multiple aetiology of restoration failure is a common occurrence

Restoration failure criteria	Causes/comments
Colour match (aesthetics)	• Important to get patients' views especially in the anterior aesthetic zone – they may or may not be concerned. • Underlying discoloration from stained dentine. • Superficial discoloration from marginal/surface staining. • Underlying discoloration from corrosion products (amalgam; see Figure 8.1). • Aged tooth-coloured restorative materials become stained and discoloured due to water absorption leading to a gradual change in optical properties (Figure 8.2).

Marginal integrity	• Loss of marginal integrity (*causing plaque retention*) caused by:
	  – Long-term creep/corrosion/ditching of amalgams (Figure 8.3)
	  – Marginal shrinkage of resin composites/bonding agent (Figure 8.4)
	  – Marginal dissolution/shrinkage of glass ionomer cements
	  – Marginal chipping under occlusal loading due to poor edge strength
	  – Presence of marginal ledges/overhangs, poor contour (Figure 8.5).
	• If the patient can keep the failed margin plaque- and recurrent caries-free and it is not of aesthetic/functional concern, then this partial loss of integrity may not be a sole cause to repair/replace the restoration.

Marginal discoloration	• Micro-/macro-defects at the tooth–restoration interface will permit exogenous stain penetration along the outer perimeter of the restoration as well as towards the pulp. • Poor aesthetics (Figure 8.6). • An indication of marginal integrity failure. • Not necessarily an indication for recurrent caries.

Loss of bulk integrity	• Restorations may be bulk fractured/partially or completely lost due to:
	  – Heavy occlusal loading – lack of occlusal analysis before restoring the tooth (Figure 8.7)
	  – Poor cavity design leading to weakened, thin-section restorations (especially for amalgams – Figure 8.8)
	  – Poor bonding technique/contamination leading to an adhesive bond failure and lack of retention.
	  – Inadequate condensation technique/curing causing intrinsic material structural weaknesses (e.g. voids, 'soggy bottom').
	• Patients will often complain of a 'hole in the tooth' where food debris is trapped – ↑ caries risk (Figure 8.9).
	• Bulk loss of restoration or occlusal wear may affect the bite/occlusal scheme (Figures 8.10, 8.11)

8

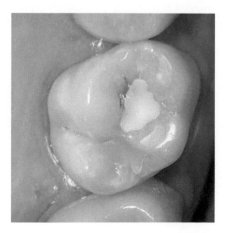

Figure 8.4 Occlusal resin composites on the UL6. Note the poor aesthetics and marginal staining/breakdown. This restoration may be replaced (due to its small size) in a high caries risk patient with poor oral hygiene, as plaque stagnation will be a problem at the defective margin.

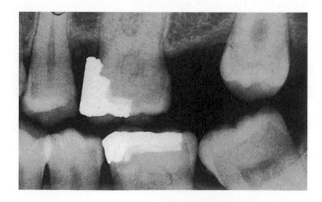

Figure 8.5 A ledged radio-opaque restoration (amalgam in this case) on the mesial aspect of UL6. Due to plaque stagnation, mesial alveolar bone loss has occurred along with radiographic evidence of caries (radiolucency beneath the overhang – care is needed to distinguish this from radiographic cervical burn-out).

Q8.5: What has caused this ledge to occur?

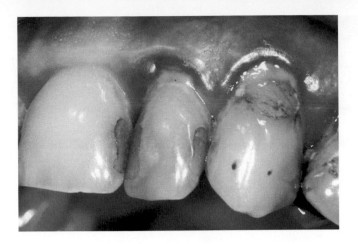

Figure 8.6 Marginal staining evident on the resin composite restorations, mesial UL1, mesial and distal UL2 and buccal cervical UL3. Patient complained of poor aesthetics. Note the plaque accumulation at the gingival margins of UL2 and UL3, posing a caries risk in these areas.

Q8.6: What periodontal condition has been caused by the accumulated plaque and what is its relevance to replacing the restorations?

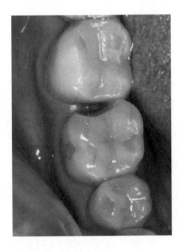

Figure 8.7 The resin composite restoration on LR6 has fractured at the distal marginal ridge due to a heavy occlusal contact with the opposing cusp.

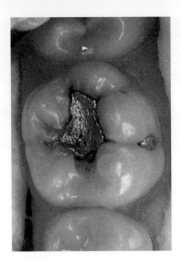

Figure 8.8 A fractured occlusal amalgam restoration in LL6.

Q8.8: What factors have resulted in this fracture?

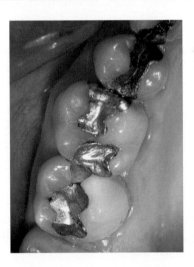

Figure 8.9 Fractured amalgam restorations UR7 mesial and UR4 distal, which need repair due to plaque stagnation and recurrent caries.

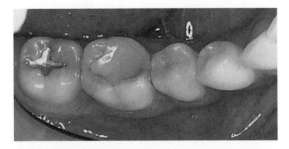

Figure 8.10 Occlusal wear on resin composite restoration LR6.

Q8.10: Does this finding necessitate the replacement of this restoration?

8

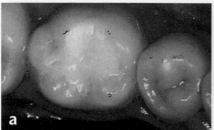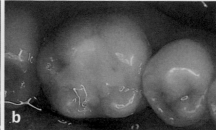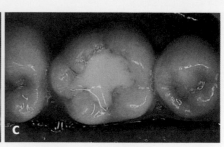

Figure 8.11 (**a**) Posterior occlusal restoration on LL6 at time of placement (blue marks on teeth are made by articulating paper checking the occlusion). (**b**) Same restoration 5 years after placement showing early signs of occlusal wear. (**c**) Restoration 9 years after placement, with further loss of occlusal definition. Margins intact and there were no symptoms from this tooth, aesthetics a little compromised – this does not constitute a restoration failure and the restoration can be monitored.

8.2.1 Aetiology

The multifactorial aetiology of restoration failure is often due to manifestations of inherent long-term weaknesses in the mechanical properties of different restorative materials (e.g. poor edge strength, wear, compressive strength, water absorption, etc.) and/or problems in the technical application of the restorative material for the chosen clinical situation (i.e. incorrect choice of material and poor placement technique).

8.2.2 Restorative material used

The physical properties of the different direct, plastic restorations at a dentist's disposal have been discussed in Chapter 6. Longevity will be affected by:

- The differences in physical properties of each material (e.g. bulk amalgam has the greatest strength and resistance to wear; glass ionomer cement (GIC) is the most soluble long term; resin composites exhibit volumetric shrinkage)

- The occlusal loading placed on individual restorations (which might cause materials to wear/fatigue/fracture more quickly than others)

- Simplicity of the clinical handling of the material (the easier it is to manipulate by the nurse/dentist and the fewer stages required for its placement, the less chance for iatrogenic weaknesses to be introduced)

- Linked to the point above, the clinical skill of the operator

- Rapid developments in dental material science. As the mechanical properties and placement techniques are continuously being developed and improved, so the longevity of new materials will surely improve.

Clinical research studies and statistical meta-analyses of past data have attempted to answer numerically the question regarding restoration longevity. However, due to the numerous uncontrollable variables mentioned (primarily the operator and the patient), obtaining a precise figure is impossible and arguably irrelevant! Often-quoted *average* age ranges of restorations at the time of replacement are:

- Amalgam restorations: 10–15 years

- Composite restorations: 5–8 years

- GIC restorations: 3–5 years.

However, this does not mean all GICs for example, will catastrophically fail after 5 years or that all amalgams will last 15 years without any problems. The hotly debated issue regarding the assessment criteria for designating failure (see next section) rears its head when considering the above longevity figures. It must be appreciated that the weighted clinical importance of some of the criteria for failure assessment (outlined in Table 8.1) will be dependent on the restorative material being assessed. For example, when considering aesthetics as an assessment of restoration failure, a black, tarnished amalgam with ditched, corroded margins on a premolar tooth may be considered functional (as it might be detrimental to the remaining tooth to replace it), whereas a mildly stained resin composite may be considered seriously for repair/replacement (as the repair procedure is relatively simple and non-destructive). Which restoration has actually 'failed'? The most useful answer to the lead question in this section is one given by an experienced operator who has monitored their own patients over many years and has seen failed restorations they were responsible for placing, appreciated the causes of failure, and then repaired/replaced them. This individual can give an honest estimate of the longevity of the restorations placed with his/her own hand, incorporating into this the individual patient factors.

8.2.3 How may restoration outcome be assessed?

There are several indices available to clinical researchers to help evaluate the causes and time lines for restoration failure made from different dental materials (USPHS, Ryge, and Hickel criteria to name but three). However, interpretation of collected data depends on what was designated a failure in the first place. A restoration's success may be judged on its clinical or radiographic appearance and form or on its function or whether the tooth is pain- or caries-free. When assessing patients in dental practice, either on primary examination or recall, the aspects of a restoration to be assessed are shown in Table 8.1. Each of the criteria can be given scores on a numerical scale depending on the degree of 'failure'. Restoration failure is mechanical in origin. However, with experience and consideration of the clinical knowledge of the patient and the patient's views, the clinician is able to make a judgement as to the degree of failure and the necessity of operative intervention, in most cases. Note that a 'failed' restoration may require replacement in one patient, but a similar 'failure' in another patient may be accepted without intervention, depending on other factors. Therefore, the decision when to replace/repair a restoration will depend on input from the experienced dentist and the patient.

8.2.4 How long should restorations last?

There are numerous factors that affect the answer to this important question that many patients will, quite reasonably, ask:

- The caries risk status of the patient (the higher the caries risk for a prolonged period of time, the less likely it is for restorations to last as long without problems usually caused by poor patient maintenance).

- The age of the patient. When clinical data from adolescents and adults are compared, restorations last longer in adults. This may reflect the susceptibility to caries of younger people or differences in attitude towards dental care.

- The type and size of restorations. Small restorations are easier to place and are easier for the patient to clean and so will last longer than larger ones.

- The restorative material used (see previous section).

- The diagnostic criteria of the dentist. This is particularly important with respect to recurrent caries, because this is the most common reason dentists give for replacing restorations (see later).

- The age of the dentist. Young dentists, with less clinical experience, tend to replace more restorations than older dentists.

- Whether the dentist is reviewing their own work or that of another dentist. Changing dentists puts a patient 'at risk' of the diagnosis of failed restorations and again, is dependent on the criteria used to define failure, but this time without any prior background clinical information.

- The care/attitude/motivation of the patient in maintaining their oral/dental health. Restorations are only ever as good as the operator placing them and the patient looking after them.

Table 8.2 Causes of tooth failure

Tooth failure		Comments
Mechanical	Enamel margin	• Poor cavity design can leave weak, unsupported/undermined enamel margins which fracture under occlusal load. • Cavity preparation techniques (burs) cause subsurface micro-cracks within the grain of enamel prisms, so weakening the surface ultrastructure (see Chapter 5, Figure 5.35). • Adhesive shrinkage stresses on prisms at enamel surface can cause them to be pulled apart causing cohesive marginal failure in tooth structure and leading to a micro-leakage risk (Figure 8.12).
	Dentine margin	• Adhesive bond to hydrophilic dentine results in a poorer quality bond which hydrolyses over time leading to ↑ risk of micro-leakage. • Deep approximal cavities often have exposed margins on dentine. Poor moisture control leads to compromised bonding technique, in turn ↑ risk of micro-leakage.
	Bulk coronal/cusp fracture	• Large restorations will weaken coronal strength of remaining hard tissue. • Loss of marginal ridges/peripheral enamel will weaken the tooth crown. • Cusps absorb oblique loading stresses and are prone to leverage/fracture (Figure 8.13). • Can cause symptoms of food-packing, sensitivity.
	Root fracture	• Often root-filled, heavily restored teeth (with post-core-crown) under heavy occlusal/lateral loads. • Traumatic injury. • Symptoms variable (pain, mobility, tenderness on biting) and radiographic assessment useful.
Biological	Recurrent caries	• New caries at a tooth–restoration gap with plaque accumulation (Figure 8.14). • Detected clinically or with radiographs. • Marginal stain is not an indicator of recurrent caries. • Can affect a section of margin and not the whole restoration.
	Pulp status	• Heavily restored teeth are more liable to pulp inflammation (Figure 8.15). • Iatrogenic damage or ongoing disease may cause pulp necrosis.
	Periodontal disease	• Examination of the periodontium required for loss of attachment, pocket depths, bone levels (Figure 8.16). • Can be exacerbated by poor marginal adaptation of restorations (causing plaque and debris stagnation)/margins encroaching into the periodontal biological width.

8

8.3 Tooth failure

Teeth can fail for *mechanical/structural* reasons and/or *biological* reasons, either together with, or independently from, restoration failure (Table 8.2).

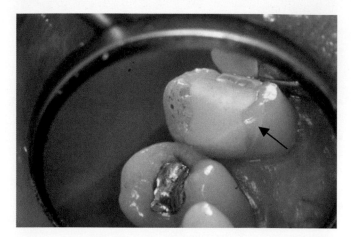

Figure 8.12 A resin composite restoration in a maxillary premolar with a fine enamel crack evident on the palatal cusp (white line) remote to the tooth–restoration interface (arrow).

Q8.12: What has caused this enamel crack?

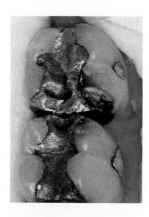

Figure 8.13 The mesiobuccal cusp of LR7 has fractured off due to excessive loading of the weakened crown and possible undermining of the cusp when the cavity was originally prepared.

Q8.13: Which coronal structural feature is missing that has contributed to the increased weakness of the remaining tooth structure?

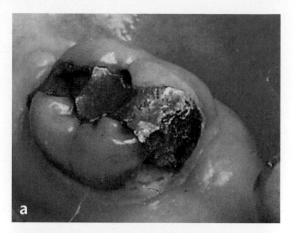

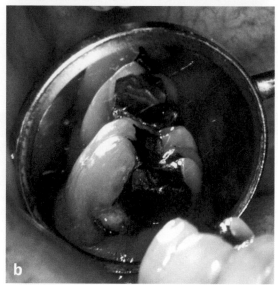

Figure 8.14 (**a**) Recurrent caries at the cervical margin gap between the tooth and amalgam in a mandibular molar. (**b**) Active, cavitated recurrent caries adjacent to an amalgam restoration with plaque retention.

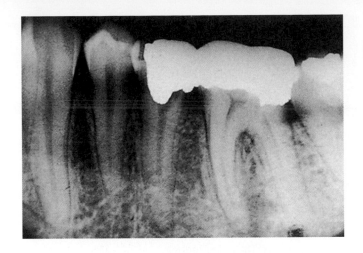

Figure 8.15 Periapical radiograph of a heavily restored LL5; over time the pulp has become non-vital and there is radiographic evidence of pulpal necrosis.

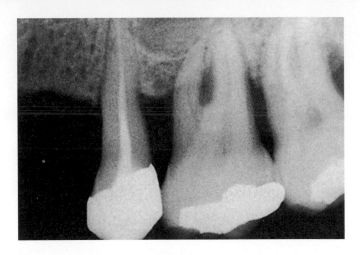

Figure 8.16 A periapical radiograph of a successful coronally restored UL6. Note the loss of alveolar bone support caused by periodontal disease leading to excessive mobility.

Q8.15i: Can you spot it?

Q8.15ii: What anatomical feature might confuse your diagnosis?

Q8.15iii: As the amalgam restoration has not extended into the pulp, why does it appear as though it has?

8.4 Monitoring the patient/course of the disease

8.4.1 Recall assessment and frequency

The recall visit follows a pattern similar to the initial assessment detailed in Chapter 2. The history will concentrate on what has happened since the dentist and patient last met. For instance, it is important to recheck the medical history carefully, but questions about past dental history need not be asked again except to check that no other dental treatment has been provided in the interim. When the clinical examination is carried out, particular attention is paid to areas noted as important or specifically requiring monitoring, e.g. caries, restorations, toothwear (see later).

8.4.2 Points to consider (especially for a previously high caries risk patient)

- Are existing restorations stable?
- Is there any clinical evidence for new lesions/demineralization?
- Is there evidence of lesion progress on radiographs (see Figure 8.17)?
- Are the dietary risk factors still present?
- Is oral bacterial balance under control?
  - Check oral hygiene (procedures and disclosing solutions)
  - Consider re-doing chairside tests (see Chapter 2)

- Has home care (topical remineralizing agents/high fluoride toothpastes, mouthwashes, etc.) helped? Has there been patient compliance?

Visual and radiographic examination may be required, with repeated bitewing radiographs every 6–12 months for high risk/caries active individuals (see Figure 8.17). If the patient has modified the causative factors and reduced their risk, becoming caries inactive, then subsequent radiographs may only be required at 18–24 month intervals, but these are only approximate guidelines and will be subject to change depending on the patient's response to treatment and preventive advice. The intervals should be judged on an individual patient basis, just like the recall frequency (Table 8.3).

8.4.3 Monitoring toothwear

As toothwear is usually an ongoing problem on first presentation at the dental surgery, it is important to be able to monitor its progress in order to see if it is getting worse, at what rate, or to see if controlling measures advised are having an effect at reducing the rate/stopping further progress. Monitoring methods may include:

- *Clinical digital photography*: standardized digital photography of the patient's teeth as shown in figures in this section, with good lighting,

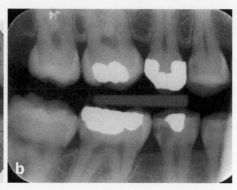

Figure 8.17 (**a**) Right bitewing radiograph of a high caries risk patient with early lesions evident distal UR4 and distal LR5. (**b**) Right bitewing radiograph of the same patient 11 months later showing significant progression of the two lesions. The caries control strategies discussed in Chapter 4 had not been fully implemented by either the dentist or the patient.

Table 8.3 Average recall frequency ranges for patients with respect to lesions present and level of caries susceptibility – note, recall frequencies must be tailored to the individual patient and the figures presented are purely a guide

Identify	Lesion			No lesion (mICDAS 0)	
	Cavitated (mICDAS 3,4)	Non-cavitated (mICDAS 1,2)			
	High risk	*High risk*	*Low risk*	*High risk (un-modifiable factors)*	*Low risk*
Recall frequency	2–6 months	3–6 months	6–12 months	3–6 months	12–18 months

Adapted from Domejean *et al*. Minimal Intervention Treatment Plan (MITP): practical implementation in general practice. *J Min Intervent Dent* 2009;**2**:103–23.

8

can be helpful for comparison over months and years. An overview can be gained from this rather than detailed measurements of any lesion change. Note, in many countries, full written consent from the patient may be required before images can be captured and stored.

- *Toothwear indices*: these are clinical scoring systems that are available to permit objective numerical scores of the degree of toothwear to be noted, reassessed, and compared at a later date. Some indices will also help with the care planning regimen required for the individual patient. Unfortunately, as with many of these indices, they are often complicated and time consuming in use. Their use in research and epidemiological studies is recommended, but in general dental practice their use may be limited.

- *Serial, dated study models* (see Figure 8.18): Casts of the dentition can be made from impressions at 12–18 month intervals in patients where the toothwear appears to be progressing, in order to be able to compare changes and develop further care plans. Again, as with clinical photography, the changes will have to be quite extensive to be noticed. The patient should be given the dated casts to keep safely and bring to future appointments. This also may help to evaluate better the attitude/motivation of the individual patient to the toothwear problem.

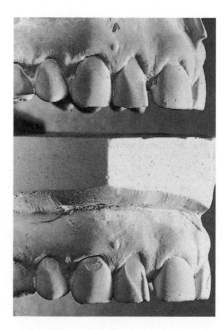

Figure 8.18 Serial study models taken with a 3-year interval showing the progress of toothwear lesions on the buccal aspects of UR234.

● *Profilometry*: Using laboratory-based laser scanners, serial models can be scanned to give accurate changes in lesion dimensions over a period of time. This is a useful research tool at present. In the future, chairside scanners will be developed to permit this detailed level of assessing changes in lesions over time to be carried out within the practice.

8.5 Repairing/replacing restorations

Modern restorations can be *repaired* or *replaced* when deemed necessary by the operator and the patient. The decision to repair or replace a restoration is one that has to be made specifically for the particular restoration in the particular patient. When significant portions of the restoration (>50%) have failed or the surrounding tooth structure is structurally and/or functionally compromised, replacement of the restoration will be indicated. In most other cases, careful repair of the deficient, fractured or weakened sections may be appropriate. When removing old restorations completely there is a significant chance of enlarging the cavity with a rotary instrument due to similarities in colour of the restoration and surrounding tooth structure. However, an alternative restorative material can then be chosen. Repairing failing portions of an existing restoration is the more conservative and minimally invasive of the two procedures, but usually uses the same restorative material as the original restoration.

8.5.1 Dental amalgam

● Relatively easy to remove remaining restoration/loose fragment. A tungsten carbide (TC) Beaver-type bur (see Figure 5.34d) is used to cut through the amalgam from its centre towards the periphery of the portion to be removed (avoiding the cavity margins). Large fragments are usually dislodged or can be flicked away using hand excavators (see Chapter 5).

● Cavity margins may be 'freshened up' using rotary instrumentation to remove stain or early demineralized hard tissues only if the restoration is to be repaired/replaced using a tooth-coloured restorative material.

● Retention has to be gained macro-mechanically via cavity undercuts, slots or grooves. If replacing the complete restoration, these retentive features will often already feature in the existing cavity design and may only need slight modification. When repairing the damaged portion of the restoration only, these retentive design features should be cut into the retained portion of the original restoration to avoid further loss and weakening of the surrounding tooth structure.

● Some may advocate the use of chemical retention, using a bonded amalgam technique, in an attempt to conserve remaining tooth structure, but there is limited evidence for the long-term success rates of this repair technique (Chapters 6, 7).

● If the above can be carried out, then the repair can be completed using amalgam. If not, chemically adhesive GIC might be the material of choice. Margins must be contoured appropriately avoiding ledges/overhangs/voids.

8.5.2 Composites/GIC

● It is more usual to repair rather than replace adhesive restorations unless there is a gross aesthetic concern. In this case, old restorations may be veneered with new material (the old restoration resurfaced with an up-to-date, shade-matched equivalent rather than replaced).

● Use rotary instrumentation to remove defective portion of restoration. Care must be taken to avoid cavity over-preparation as it can be difficult to distinguish between the adhesive restoration and cavity margin due to colour similarities. Air-abrasive techniques using alumina or bioactive glass powders might facilitate this process due to their inherent selectivity for resin composites and/or grossly demineralized enamel.

● Fresh cavity margins should expose a reduced surface energy and roughened enamel and/or dentine surface for better micro-mechanical/chemical adhesion.

– *GIC*: condition all surfaces with 10% polyacrylic acid for 10 seconds, wash thoroughly, blot dry and apply/pack GIC (with matrixing as appropriate).

– *Composite*: acid-etch with 37% orthophosphoric acid for 20 seconds (enamel) and 10 seconds (dentine), wash thoroughly, and dry briefly. Silanating agent may be used to couple new methacrylate-based composite resins to old (painted on the bonding surface of the old restoration and evaporated), dentine bonding agent applied onto cavity surfaces and gently dried (depending on which type is used), light-cured and then composite added in small increments, cured, and finished. Often the silanating agent may be omitted as it can interfere with the adhesive chemistry of the dentine bonding agent and it may be clinically difficult to separate these two procedures.

8

8.6 Answers to self-test questions

Q8.1: What restorative material should be used to replace this amalgam?

A: Dental composite.

Q8.2: What would be the difficulty faced by the dentist when replacing this Class III restoration?

A: Aesthetics: matching the natural translucency from the incisal edge through to the mesial aspect of the UL2. An aesthetic layered composite restoration would have to be placed carefully mimicking the underlying dentine and overlying enamel shades.

Q8.5: What has caused this ledge to occur?

A: A poorly adapted/wedged matrix band at the cervical margin of the approximal Class II cavity.

Q8.6: What periodontal condition has been caused by the accumulated plaque and what is its relevance to replacing the restorations?

A: Chronic marginal gingivitis. This would need to be remedied with improved oral hygiene techniques prior to any restoration being placed in order to ensure optimal moisture control during placement of the new composite restorations.

Q8.8: What factors have resulted in this fracture?

A: Poor cavity design: the mesial portion of the cavity was too shallow and the amalgam fractured under occlusal load due to its inherent weakness in thin section and lack of macro-mechanical retentive features; inappropriate choice of material: a resin composite may have been a better choice, so preventing any unnecessary extension of the cavity.

Q8.10: Does this finding necessitate the replacement of this restoration?

A: No. The restoration is fully functional and is not causing any clinical problems.

Q8.12: What has caused this enamel crack?

A: Caused by shrinkage stress from the composite pulling on the prismatic enamel structure and causing cohesive failure in the enamel.

Q8.13: Which coronal structural feature is missing that has contributed to the increased weakness of the remaining tooth structure?

A: A missing mesial marginal ridge.

Q8.15i: Can you spot it?

A: Widening of the periodontal ligament space at the root apex with loss of lamina dura in this area of the LL5.

Q8.15ii: What anatomical feature might confuse your diagnosis?

A: An overlying mental foramen.

Q8.15iii: As the amalgam restoration has not extended into the pulp, why does it appear as though it has?

A: There is an additional buccal cervical amalgam restoration, the radiographic opacity of which has superimposed itself over the pulp chamber radiolucency.

8

Appendix: Further Information

The contents of this book should be digested along with equivalent recommended texts in periodontology, prosthodontics, endodontics, radiology and radiography, oral biology, and dental anatomy and histology. The authors made a conscious decision not to include a bibliography at the end of each chapter in this edition of *Pickard's Manual of Operative Dentistry*. It was felt that the clinical and research evidence base for those aspects of operative dentistry discussed in this text has been expanding rapidly in recent years and will continue to do so. Any list provided will soon be out of date and not necessarily relevant to contemporary dental practice.

Instead, it was decided to provide information on some specialist reference texts in certain subject areas to permit the reader to gain more in-depth knowledge, e.g. in caries and dental materials science. Also, a list of selected keywords and phrases have been supplied for use in popular internet search engines. Again, these have been suggested in order to offer the interested reader a further insight into subject areas, while complementing the content of this book. It is hoped this system will offer up-to-date sources of information which will be automatically updated as future research is published. Care must be taken when interpreting any information gleaned from open-access platforms as their origins or validity may not be verifiable or even correct. One useful academic search engine for validated, peer-reviewed citations is PubMed:

http://www.ncbi.nlm.nih.gov/sites/entrez?db=pubmed

Reference texts

- Andreasen JO, Andreasen FM, Andersson L. (eds) (2007) *Textbook and colour atlas of traumatic injuries to teeth*, 4th edn. Oxford: Blackwell Munksgaard.
  http://eu.wiley.com/WileyCDA/WileyTitle/productCd-1405129549.html

- Fejerskov O, Kidd EAM. (eds) (2008) *Dental caries: the disease and its clinical management*. Oxford: Blackwell Munksgaard.
  http://eu.wiley.com/WileyCDA/WileyTitle/productCd-1405138890,descCd-tableOfContents.html

- Darvell BW. (2009) *Material science for dentistry*, 9th edn. Cambridge: Woodhead CRC Press.
  http://www.woodheadpublishing.com/en/book.aspx?bookID=1547

- Curtis RV, Watson TF. (eds) (2008) *Dental biomaterials: imaging, testing and modelling*. Cambridge: Woodhead CRC Press.
  http://www.woodheadpublishing.com/en/book.aspx?bookID=1347

- Department of Health. (2009) *Delivering better oral health. An evidence-based toolkit for prevention – second edition*. London: Department of Health/BASCD.
  http://www.dh.gov.uk/en/Publicationsand statistics/Publications/PublicationsPolicyAndGuidance/DH_102331

Keywords/phrases

- **Chapter 1**: Sjögren's syndrome; xerostomia; Maillard reaction and caries; dentine matrix metalloproteinases (MMPs); toothwear; GORD and dental symptoms; hereditary dental conditions.

- **Chapter 2**: ICDAS; cariogram

- **Chapter 3**: Basic Erosive Wear Examination (BEWE); Smith and Knight toothwear index.

- **Chapter 4**: dental remineralizing solutions; CPP-ACP.

- **Chapter 5**: BDA infection control (UK); dental infection control Department of Health (UK); HTM01-05; minimal intervention dentistry; minimally invasive dentistry; glossary of prosthodontic terms.

- **Chapter 8**: dental restoration failure; dental restoration longevity.

Index

Note to index: In most cases, the word 'dental' has been omitted; for example, caries; occlusion; pain